Updates in Clinical Dermatology

Updates in Clinical Dermatology aims to promote the rapid and efficient transfer of medical research into clinical practice. It is published in four volumes per year. Covering new developments and innovations in all fields of clinical dermatology, it provides the clinician with a review and summary of recent research and its implications for clinical practice. Each volume is focused on a clinically relevant topic and explains how research results impact diagnostics, treatment options and procedures as well as patient management. The reader-friendly volumes are highly structured with core messages, summaries, tables, diagrams and illustrations and are written by internationally well-known experts in the field. A volume editor supervises the authors in his/her field of expertise in order to ensure that each volume provides cutting-edge information most relevant and useful for clinical dermatologists. Contributions to the series are peer reviewed by an editorial board.

Esraa M. AlEdani • Howard Maibach
Editors

COVID-19 Vaccination and Dermatological Diseases

Springer

Editors
Esraa M. AlEdani
University of Basrah-Medical Faculty
Basrah, Iraq

Howard Maibach
School of Medicine
University of California, San Francisco
San Francisco, CA, USA

ISSN 2523-8884 ISSN 2523-8892 (electronic)
Updates in Clinical Dermatology
ISBN 978-3-031-87790-2 ISBN 978-3-031-87791-9 (eBook)
https://doi.org/10.1007/978-3-031-87791-9

This Springer imprint is published by the registered company Springer Nature Switzerland AG
The registered company address is: Gewerbestrasse 11, 6330 Cham, Switzerland

Preface

A new chapter in medical science has been created by the convergence of dermatology and the COVID-19 pandemic, highlighting the significant influence of worldwide health emergencies on skin-related disorders and their treatment. The complex interaction between COVID-19, its vaccine, and different dermatological disorders is examined in this book, which offers a thorough examination of the ways in which a respiratory virus and its immune-mediated effects might affect skin health.

Each chapter explores the particular difficulties brought on by the epidemic, ranging from the treatment of skin cancer to autoimmune diseases like lupus and psoriasis. New patterns of disease presentation, aggravation, and recovery in dermatology have been influenced by the interruption of normal care, the immunological dysregulation brought on by SARS-CoV-2, and the extraordinary deployment of COVID-19 vaccinations.

The human element—patients' experiences, the robustness of healthcare systems, and the role of innovation, such as telemedicine, in guaranteeing continuity of care—is highlighted in this study in addition to the scientific and clinical components. This book attempts to educate and direct dermatologists, researchers, and other healthcare professionals in negotiating the changing terrain of dermatological care during and after the pandemic by synthesizing case reports, research, and expert insights.

This book is a testament to the value of flexibility, teamwork, and knowledge acquisition in overcoming obstacles and enhancing patient outcomes in dermatology as we continue to learn from these extraordinary times.

Basrah, Iraq — Esraa M. AlEdani
San Francisco, CA, USA — Howard Maibach

Contents

Overview of COVID-19 and Its Vaccination and Its Relation to Dermatology

1

Esraa M. AlEdani

The world economy, medical sciences, and health have all been significantly impacted by the COVID-19 pandemic. Since its initial appearance in late 2019, COVID-19, which is caused by the unique SARS-CoV-2 virus, has sparked an unprecedented global response that includes the quick production and distribution of vaccinations. COVID-19 has demonstrated extensive systemic effects, including noteworthy dermatological consequences, in addition to its respiratory manifestations. With an emphasis on the disease's cutaneous signs, vaccine-related dermatological reactions, and the function of skin as a marker of systemic involvement, this chapter examines the relationship between COVID-19 and dermatology.

1.1 COVID-19: An Overview

A virus that mostly affects the respiratory system, COVID-19 is extremely contagious. Nonetheless, a variety of clinical manifestations, such as neurological, gastrointestinal, dermatological, and cardiovascular problems, have resulted from its systemic nature. The spike protein of the virus enters host cells through the ACE2 receptor, which is expressed in the skin and other tissues.

Skin signs have drawn attention as possible early markers of COVID-19 or as part of the systemic involvement in severe cases, even if respiratory symptoms such fever, cough, and shortness of breath predominate the clinical picture [1].

1.2 COVID-19 Vaccination: A Global Milestone

The mainstay of international efforts to stop the spread of COVID-19 has been vaccination. A notable scientific accomplishment has been the quick development of vaccines, such as those based on mRNA (Pfizer-BioNTech, Moderna), adenoviral vectors (AstraZeneca, Johnson & Johnson), and inactivated viruses (Sinovac, Sinopharm).

The growing use of vaccines has raised awareness of a number of side effects, including dermatological problems, even though they have been essential in lowering the severity and death of disease. For immunologists and dermatologists, these cutaneous reactions are essential because they reveal information about how the immune system is responding to the vaccination [2].

E. M. AlEdani (✉)
University of Basrah-Medical Faculty, Basrah, Iraq

E. M. AlEdani, H. Maibach (eds.), *COVID-19 Vaccination and Dermatological Diseases*, Updates in Clinical Dermatology, https://doi.org/10.1007/978-3-031-87791-9_1

1.3 Cutaneous Manifestations of COVID-19

COVID-19-related cutaneous symptoms can be divided into multiple categories:

- Exanthems: Morbilliform rash that resembles drug-induced responses or measles.
- Vascular lesions include retiform purpura linked to coagulopathy, livedo reticularis, and chillblain-like (COVID toes).
- Urticarial eruptions are frequently associated with the initial phases of infection.
- Vesicular eruptions: May indicate direct viral involvement, as they resemble varicella (chickenpox).

Particularly in patients with unusual presentations or no symptoms, these dermatological features are essential for early diagnosis [3].

1.4 Dermatological Reactions to COVID-19 Vaccination

Although usually modest, post-vaccination dermatological symptoms are becoming more widely acknowledged. These may consist of:

- Localized erythema, edema, or pain at the injection site are examples of injection site responses. Days after vaccination.
- Delayed hypersensitivity responses, commonly referred to as "COVID arm," manifest as itchy, erythematous plaques.
- Rarely, urticaria and angioedema are symptoms of a systemic allergic reaction.
- Pre-existing problems getting worse: instances where vaccinations cause or worsen autoimmune blistering disorders like Bullous Pemphigoid, psoriasis, or eczema.

Clinicians must comprehend these reactions in order to differentiate between less serious side effects that call for intervention and benign vaccine-related side effects [4].

1.5 The Immune System and Dermatological Link

The immune system is impacted by COVID-19 and its vaccines in ways that affect dermatological health:

- In patients with preexisting autoimmune disorders, inflammatory skin illnesses may be a manifestation of immunological dysregulation caused by COVID-19.
- Immune responses to vaccinations can sometimes be strong and trigger flare-ups of autoimmune diseases or the advent of new disorders like vitiligo or lupus.

These findings highlight how crucial it is to comprehend the fine line that separates protective immunity from immunological overreaction in dermatology [5].

1.6 Understanding Cutaneous Signs as Diagnostic Clues

Being the largest organ in the body, the skin frequently reflects interior functions. Skin symptoms of COVID-19 could be used as early diagnostic markers or gauges of the severity of the illness. For example:

Often seen in younger, otherwise healthy people, chillblain-like lesions (also known as "COVID toes") are believed to be caused by immune-mediated inflammation or microvascular damage.

Acrocyanosis and liver reticularis are vascular patterns that may indicate coagulopathies, which are common side effects in severe COVID-19 cases.

Children's multisystem inflammatory syndrome (MIS-C): This post-infectious consequence highlights the skin's involvement in systemic inflammatory disorders by presenting with skin signs like rash and mucocutaneous involvement.

Dermatologists can help with early detection by identifying these patterns, especially in patients who do not exhibit the typical respiratory symptoms of COVID-19 [5].

1.7 Post-COVID Dermatological Conditions

Dermatological sequelae, a phenomena linked to long-term COVID or post-acute sequelae of SARS-CoV-2 infection (PASC), have also been linked to the aftermath of COVID-19 infection. These consist of:

Persistent hair loss: As a result of the physiological stress brought on by COVID-19, telogen effluvium, a type of diffuse hair shedding, has been extensively documented.

Dermatitis and persistent urticaria: Immune dysregulation following an infection may show up as a flare-up of pre-existing inflammatory skin diseases or persistent hives.

Pigmentary changes: As a result of chronic inflammation or scarring, some patients experience hyperpigmentation or hypopigmentation in the locations of prior lesions.

Giving recuperating patients complete care requires an understanding of their long-term repercussions [6].

1.8 Vaccine-Induced Dermatological Reactions: Immune Mechanisms

The decrease in severe illness and death has been largely attributed to the immunological response that COVID-19 vaccinations have induced. But it has also led to a variety of dermatological responses, which can be broadly categorized as follows:

- Immediate hypersensitivity reactions: Although uncommon, urticaria, angioedema, and anaphylaxis must be identified and treated very away.
- Slow responses: appearing at the injection site as itchy nodules, papules, or erythematous plaques. Despite being annoying, these reactions usually go away on their own.
- Autoimmune skin illnesses include lupus, dermatomyositis, and autoimmune blistering diseases, as well as those that are newly diagnosed or worsened. The method frequently entails autoreactive T-cell bystander activation or molecular mimicry.
- Vasculitis: Vaccine administration has been connected to cases of small-vessel vasculitis, highlighting the necessity of close observation in vulnerable people [6].

1.9 The Role of Dermatology in Vaccine Safety and Hesitancy

Vaccine reluctance, which is partially caused by worries about adverse effects, has been one of the campaign's obstacles. Dermatologists are essential in resolving these issues since they:

- Giving precise information teaching patients that the majority of dermatological reactions are usually benign and only last temporarily.
- Finding those who are at risk: assessing for autoimmune diseases, previous allergic responses, or vaccination component sensitivities in order to reduce risks.
- Handling skin problems brought on by vaccinations: providing efficient remedies for mild to moderate allergies and working with immunologists and allergists for more severe situations.

In addition to helping to increase immunization rates, this proactive strategy can boost patient confidence in vaccination programs [6].

1.10 The Future of Dermatology in the Post-COVID Era

Opportunities for multidisciplinary study and practice have been made possible by the inclusion of dermatology in the larger framework of COVID-19 management. Future research priorities include:

- Finding cutaneous biomarkers that anticipate complications or correlate with the severity of a disease is known as biomarker discovery.
- Long-term research on the effects of vaccines: knowing how long vaccine-induced dermatological disorders last and how often they return.
- International cooperation: exchanging information on uncommon or unique manifestations of dermatological findings linked to COVID-19 in order to improve our collective understanding.
- Dermatology can maintain its crucial role in tackling the complex issues presented by COVID-19 by giving priority to these research areas [6].

1.11 Conclusion

The interdependence of several medical specializations has been highlighted by the COVID-19 pandemic, with dermatology emerging as a crucial element in comprehending and treating the disease's systemic consequences. Dermatologists have improved patient outcomes and public health initiatives by managing vaccine-related responses and detecting cutaneous symptoms of the virus. The knowledge gathered by researching COVID-19 and its vaccines will continue to influence dermatological practice as the globe enters a post-pandemic period, promoting a better comprehension of the skin's function in systemic health and illness.

This chapter lays the groundwork for more comprehensive approaches to patient care by emphasizing the value of seeing dermatology as a window into the larger physiological processes rather than in isolation.

References

1. Fernandes Q, Inchakalody VP, Merhi M, Mestiri S, Taib N, Moustafa Abo El-Ella D, Bedhiafi T, Raza A, Al Zaidan L, Mohsen MO, Yousuf Al-Nesr MA, Hssain AA, Yassine HM, Bachmann MF, Uddin S, Dermime S. Emerging COVID-19 variants and their impact on SARS-CoV-2 diagnosis, therapeutics and vaccines. Ann Med. 2022;54(1):524–40. https://doi.org/10.1080/07853890.2022.2031274. PMID: 35132910; PMCID: PMC8843115.
2. Nakashima C, Kato M, Otsuka A. Cutaneous manifestations of COVID-19 and COVID-19 vaccination. J Dermatol. 2023;50(3):280–9. https://doi.org/10.1111/1346-8138.16651. Epub 2023 Jan 13.
3. Wang C, Rademaker M, Tate B, Baker C, Foley P. SARS-CoV-2 (COVID-19) vaccination in dermatology patients on immunomodulatory and biologic agents: recommendations from the Australasian Medical Dermatology Group. Australas J Dermatol. 2021;62(2):151–6. https://doi.org/10.1111/ajd.13593. Epub 2021 Mar 30. PMID: 33786833; PMCID: PMC8250550.
4. Wack S, Patton T, Ferris LK. COVID-19 vaccine safety and efficacy in patients with immune-mediated inflammatory disease: Review of available evidence. J Am Acad Dermatol. 2021;85(5):1274–84. https://doi.org/10.1016/j.jaad.2021.07.054. Epub 2021 Aug 4. PMID: 34363909; PMCID: PMC8336973.
5. Gambichler T, Boms S, Susok L, Dickel H, Finis C, Abu Rached N, Barras M, Stücker M, Kasakovski D. Cutaneous findings following COVID-19 vaccination: review of world literature and own experience. J Eur Acad Dermatol Venereol. 2022;36(2):172–80. https://doi.org/10.1111/jdv.17744. Epub 2021 Nov 2. PMID: 34661927; PMCID: PMC8656409.
6. Aryanian Z, Ehsani A, Razavi Z, Hamzelou S, Mohseni Afshar Z, Hatami P. The COVID-19 pandemic and its impact on esthetic dermatology. J Cosmet Dermatol. 2022;21(12):6557–61. https://doi.org/10.1111/jocd.15386. Epub 2022 Sep 26. PMID: 36106524; PMCID: PMC9538429.

The Effect of COVID-19 on Acne Exacerbation

2

Mustafa Abrar Zaman and Esraa M. AlEdani

2.1 Introduction to COVID-19 and Skin Health

The COVID-19 pandemic has had a profound impact on numerous aspects of healthcare, including dermatology, resulting in significant changes in skin health and the management of skin conditions. The cutaneous manifestations linked to COVID-19 have become a crucial area of research, as they present a wide range of skin reactions that can serve as potential indicators of the severity and progression of the disease. These skin reactions can be broadly classified into two categories: those that resemble viral exanthems and those caused by systemic complications such as vasculitis or thrombotic events [1]. While the understanding of these dermatological symptoms is still in its early stages, ongoing studies aim to uncover the mechanisms driving these reactions and their broader clinical implications. A systematic review has identified a variety of skin manifestations associated with COVID-19, including maculopapular rashes, vesicular lesions, urticaria-like eruptions, and chilblains [2]. These changes in the skin can occur at various points in the disease's course, and in some cases, they may even appear before more well-known symptoms like fever or cough [2]. This has raised important questions regarding the potential diagnostic value of these cutaneous signs, with some research indicating they could serve as early warning signs of COVID-19 infection [3]. Furthermore, the frequency of these skin conditions appears to differ across different populations and regions, underscoring the need for more extensive epidemiological studies [4].

The pandemic has also dramatically altered dermatology practices, particularly in outpatient settings. Many clinics saw a sharp decrease in patient visits due to lockdown restrictions and concerns about virus transmission. This drop in appointments led to a backlog of patients suffering from worsening dermatological conditions [5, 6]. This decrease in patient volume has been linked to a rise in acute dermatological problems, such as irritant contact dermatitis and exacerbations of chronic conditions like psoriasis [5]. In response, teledermatology has become a primary method for continuing care while reducing infection risk [7, 8]. However, there is still ongoing debate about the effectiveness of teledermatology in managing more complex skin conditions. Beyond the physical effects on skin health, the pandemic has also taken a toll on the mental health of both dermatology practitioners and their patients. The stress of the pandemic, combined

M. A. Zaman (✉)
St. George's University, True Blue, Grenada

Northumbria University, Newcastle upon Tyne, UK
e-mail: mzaman5@sgu.edu,
mustafa.zaman@northumbria.ac.uk

E. M. AlEdani
University of Basrah-Medical Faculty, Basrah, Iraq

E. M. AlEdani, H. Maibach (eds.), *COVID-19 Vaccination and Dermatological Diseases*, Updates in Clinical Dermatology, https://doi.org/10.1007/978-3-031-87791-9_2

with the challenges of adapting to new practice methods, has impacted the well-being of dermatology residents and professionals [9, 10]. The potential impact of these mental health challenges on the quality of care provided to patients is an area that requires further exploration, especially as healthcare systems continue to cope with the pandemic's long-term effects. In parallel, there has been a surge in clinical trials and research focusing on the dermatological implications of COVID-19 [11, 12]. This increased research activity is critical to understanding the long-term effects of the virus on skin health and developing effective treatment protocols. The findings from these studies will likely shape future clinical guidelines, improving the overall management of skin conditions in the COVID-19 context.

As the pandemic evolves, dermatologists must remain vigilant in identifying and addressing the wide array of skin manifestations linked to COVID-19. This involves not only recognizing the clinical characteristics of these dermatological symptoms but also understanding the broader impact of the pandemic on dermatology practices and patient care. While telemedicine has proven beneficial in maintaining care, it is essential that ongoing training and education are provided to healthcare professionals to ensure that patients continue to receive comprehensive and effective treatment. The pandemic's effects on skin health have highlighted a complex interaction between the virus and dermatological conditions. The emergence of diverse skin manifestations emphasizes the need for continued research and heightened awareness within the dermatology field. As healthcare systems adjust to the challenges posed by COVID-19, the mental health and well-being of dermatology practitioners should be prioritized, alongside ensuring that patients receive prompt and effective treatment for their skin conditions.

Learning Objectives

1. Understand the impact of COVID-19 on dermatological conditions, particularly acne exacerbation, and the role of stress, lifestyle changes, and mask usage.
2. Identify the common cutaneous manifestations of COVID-19 and their potential diagnostic value as early indicators of the disease.
3. Analyze the pathophysiology of acne vulgaris, including hormonal, microbial, genetic, and environmental factors contributing to its development and severity.
4. Explore the influence of psychological factors, particularly stress, on acne exacerbation during the pandemic and the role of the hypothalamic-pituitary-adrenal (HPA) axis.
5. Evaluate the effectiveness of teledermatology in managing acne and other dermatological conditions during the pandemic, while recognizing its limitations in complex cases.
6. Examine the interplay between mental health and dermatological conditions, focusing on how stress and anxiety during the pandemic have worsened skin disorders like acne.
7. Discuss the integrated management approach for acne during COVID-19, including traditional treatments, psychological interventions, and lifestyle modifications.

2.2 Pathophysiology of Acne

Acne vulgaris is a common skin disorder marked by persistent inflammation of the pilosebaceous unit, which encompasses hair follicles and sebaceous glands. The development of acne is complex and influenced by a combination of hormonal, genetic, environmental, and microbial factors. Gaining a deep understanding of these mechanisms is essential for creating effective treatment approaches and managing this widespread condition. The primary factors contributing to acne's onset include excess sebum production (hyperseborrhea), irregular shedding of skin cells (abnormal keratinization), and the overgrowth of *Cutibacterium acnes* (formerly *Propionibacterium acnes*), a bacterium found on the skin [13, 14]. Hyperseborrhea is driven by increased sebum production, which is influenced by hormones like testosterone and dehydroepiandrosterone (DHEA). These androgens stimulate sebaceous glands, leading to excessive sebum release [15]. Fluctuations in hormone levels, particularly during puberty and the menstrual cycle, are known to aggravate acne, as multiple studies have shown a clear link between hormonal changes and acne severity [16, 17].

In addition to hormone-related factors, abnormal keratinization in hair follicles plays a critical role in acne. When keratinocytes (the cells in hair follicles) fail to shed properly and accumulate, they cause clogged pores. This blockage not only results in the formation of comedones (the hallmark lesions of acne) but also creates an environment conducive to the growth of *C. acnes*. This bacterium thrives in the oxygen-poor environment inside blocked follicles, where it contributes to inflammation, leading to the formation of papules, pustules, and other inflammatory lesions [18, 19]. The inflammatory response in acne is complex and involves various immune mechanisms. *C. acnes* stimulates the activation of the body's innate immune system, leading to the release of pro-inflammatory chemicals like cytokines and chemokines that draw immune cells to the affected area [20]. The Th1 and Th17 immune responses are particularly implicated in acne inflammation, emphasizing the role of adaptive immunity in this process [21]. Moreover, the presence of B cells in acne lesions suggests that both humoral (antibody-mediated) and cellular immune responses work together to sustain inflammation [22].

Genetics also significantly influence acne. Research has revealed certain gene variations associated with acne severity, indicating that genetic factors can affect everything from sebum production to follicular keratinization and the body's inflammatory responses [23]. Furthermore, metabolic factors, including insulin resistance, are linked to acne, with studies showing that insulin and insulin-like growth factor-1 (IGF-1) can exacerbate both sebum production and follicular hyperkeratinization [24]. Diet also plays a role, with high-glycemic-index foods and dairy products potentially worsening acne by impacting insulin levels and hormonal balance [25]. Stress is another key contributor, as psychological stress can trigger the release of neuropeptides, which in turn can heighten inflammation and sebum production, exacerbating acne symptoms [26]. The interaction between stress, hormonal changes, and immune responses creates a vicious cycle, making acne more challenging to manage. By understanding this multifaceted interplay of factors, healthcare professionals can devise more targeted treatments, addressing both the underlying causes and symptoms of acne to improve patient outcomes.

2.3 Acne Exacerbation During COVID-19

The COVID-19 pandemic has significantly affected a wide range of health conditions, including dermatological concerns like acne. Stress, lifestyle changes, and the psychological toll of the pandemic have played a crucial role in influencing skin health, especially in individuals already prone to acne. The heightened stress levels brought about by the pandemic are linked to the worsening of pre-existing conditions like acne vulgaris. This is largely due to the activation of the hypothalamic-pituitary-adrenal (HPA) axis, which raises cortisol levels in the body. Increased cortisol can lead to greater sebum production, a well-established factor in the development of acne [27, 28]. Additionally, shifts in personal hygiene habits and the frequent use of face masks during the pandemic have given rise to a condition known as "maskne." The occlusion caused by masks creates a warm and humid environment that encourages the growth of acne-causing bacteria, thereby aggravating pre-existing acne conditions. Numerous reports have documented this phenomenon, underscoring the need for dermatological awareness and new management strategies during the pandemic [29].

The psychological challenges brought on by the pandemic, such as anxiety and depression, have further exacerbated skin conditions like acne, making it even more difficult to manage these issues [30, 31]. The presence of comorbidities in individuals with pre-existing skin conditions is also worth noting. Those with conditions like acne may see their symptoms worsen due to the systemic inflammatory responses triggered by COVID-19. This can

Table 2.1 Comparison of pre-pandemic and pandemic dermatology practices

Aspect of practice	Pre-pandemic	During pandemic
Patient volume	High	Significantly reduced due to lockdowns and safety measures [5]
Mode of consultation	In-person consultations	Shift to teledermatology (video, apps) [7]
Treatment approaches	Mostly in-clinic procedures and prescriptions	Remote consultations, limited in-person interactions [6]
Follow-up rates	High follow-up rate for chronic conditions	Lower follow-up, reliance on digital consultations [9]

lead to an increase in acne lesions [32, 33]. Furthermore, medications used to treat COVID-19, such as corticosteroids, can alter skin barrier function and boost sebum production, further contributing to acne flare-ups [34, 35]. Beyond the direct effects of the virus on skin health, the pandemic has disrupted healthcare access, delaying treatment for many acne sufferers. Although telemedicine has provided some continuity in care, it cannot fully replace the need for in-person consultations, especially for severe cases of acne [36].

The combined psychological strain of the pandemic and restricted access to dermatological care has left many patients feeling frustrated and dissatisfied, which negatively affects their mental health and overall well-being [2]. Research during the pandemic has increasingly focused on the connection between mental health and skin conditions. Studies show that individuals with acne are more vulnerable to negative psychological outcomes, such as low self-esteem and social anxiety, particularly during stressful times [37]. The visibility of acne can lead to social stigmatization, a problem made worse by the isolation resulting from lockdowns and social distancing measures [38, 39]. These findings highlight the importance of an integrated approach to care that addresses both the physical and psychological dimensions of acne management during and beyond the pandemic [40]. Moreover, the rise in social media usage during the pandemic has also impacted perceptions of beauty and skin health. The portrayal of flawless skin on these platforms can create unrealistic beauty standards, leading to body image concerns and worsening the psychological burden of acne [41]. This highlights the importance of promoting realistic beauty standards and encouraging resilience among those dealing with acne during these challenging times [42] (Table 2.1).

2.4 Management of Acne Exacerbated by COVID-19

The management of acne, particularly worsened by the effects of COVID-19, has emerged as a pressing issue. The pandemic has triggered heightened stress, disrupted skincare routines, and led to the frequent use of face masks, all of which are contributing factors to acne flare-ups. One of the key contributors to acne aggravation during this period is the rise in stress and anxiety levels among individuals. It is well established that stress can worsen acne by impacting hormonal pathways, particularly increasing androgen levels, which in turn elevate sebum production and promote acne formation [43]. A systematic review has underscored the psychological toll of the pandemic, indicating that higher anxiety and stress levels can exacerbate pre-existing skin conditions, including acne [44]. As a result, psychological interventions such as cognitive behavioral therapy (CBT) and mindfulness techniques may be helpful in managing acne linked to stress [45].

Alongside psychological care, traditional topical and systemic treatments remain essential for managing acne during the pandemic. Standard topical treatments like retinoids, benzoyl peroxide, and salicylic acid are effective in reducing acne by enhancing cell turnover and curbing inflammation [46]. For more severe

Table 2.2 Summary of acne treatment modalities during COVID-19

Modality	Description	Challenges during COVID-19	Effectiveness
Topical treatments	Benzoyl peroxide, retinoids, salicylic acid	May cause irritation under face masks	High effectiveness for mild to moderate acne [49]
Systemic treatments	Antibiotics, hormonal therapies, oral retinoids	Requires regular monitoring, harder to implement with telemedicine	High effectiveness for severe acne [10]
Psychological interventions	CBT, stress management techniques	Teletherapy is accessible but lacks in-person support	Moderate to high depending on patient adherence [27]
Lifestyle changes	Diet, exercise, skincare routine	Pandemic has disrupted routines, making consistency harder	High when sustained over time [44] [25]

cases, systemic treatments such as antibiotics (e.g., doxycycline) and hormonal therapies (e.g., oral contraceptives) may be employed (Fu). The choice of treatment should be individualized, particularly in light of mask-related skin sensitivities, and should be combined with gentle skincare practices [45]. In response to the pandemic, the landscape of dermatological care has adapted significantly, with telemedicine rising as a prominent mode of patient consultation. This transition allows individuals to continue receiving acne care without needing in-person visits, which is especially beneficial for those reluctant to visit healthcare settings during the pandemic [47]. Teledermatology has proven effective in managing various skin conditions, including acne, by providing timely medical advice and prescriptions remotely [46]. In addition, lifestyle adjustments play an important role in managing acne exacerbated by the pandemic. A consistent skincare routine that includes gentle cleansing and moisturizing can help mitigate breakouts. Furthermore, dietary changes—specifically a diet rich in antioxidants and low in high-glycemic foods—can influence acne severity [48]. Incorporating regular physical activity and ensuring adequate sleep are also crucial, as these factors promote overall well-being and can reduce stress-related acne [39].Managing acne in the context of COVID-19 requires a comprehensive, multidimensional approach. This includes addressing psychological health, employing tailored pharmacological treatments, utilizing telemedicine for remote care, and making lifestyle changes. By integrating these strategies, healthcare providers can offer well-rounded, effective care for patients facing acne exacerbations during these unprecedented times (Table 2.2).

2.5 Conclusion

The COVID-19 pandemic has had a significant impact on skin health, especially for those who are prone to acne. The combination of altered lifestyles, increased stress levels, and the increasing use of face masks has made acne, a common dermatological ailment, worse. Higher sebum production has been linked to increased stress through hormonal pathways, and the use of masks has fostered an environment that is favourable to the development of acne. The severity of acne has been exacerbated by the psychological effects of the pandemic, such as increased anxiety and depression. This emphasises the need for integrated care approaches that address mental and physical health. During the pandemic, acne management calls for a diversified strategy. Conventional therapies that continue to be effective include benzoyl peroxide, topical retinoids, and systemic therapies. Nonetheless, the increasing use of teledermatology has turned into an indispensable tool for continuing patient care while lowering the risk of infection. Furthermore, lifestyle adjustments such as stress reduction, diet, and regular skincare practices are essential in reducing the severity of acne flare-ups. Prioritising holistic care that promotes patients' psychological and dermatological well-being is crucial as the pandemic continues to strain healthcare systems.

References

1. Kaya G, Kaya A, Saurat J. Clinical and histopathological features and potential pathological mechanisms of skin lesions in COVID-19: review of the literature. Dermatopathology. 2020.
2. Jamshidi P, Hajikhani B, Mirsaeidi M, Vahidnezhad H, Dadashi M, Nasiri MJ. Skin manifestations in COVID-19 patients: are they indicators for disease severity? A systematic review. Front Med. 2021.
3. Visconti A, Bataille V, Rossi N, Kluk J, Murphy R, Puig S, et al. Diagnostic value of cutaneous manifestation of SARS-CoV-2 infection. Br J Dermatol. 2021.
4. Sameni F, Hajikhani B, Yaslianifard S, Goudarzi M, Owlia P, Nasiri MJ, et al. COVID-19 and skin manifestations: an overview of case reports/case series and meta-analysis of prevalence studies. Front Med. 2020;7.
5. Yim K, Yim RM, Gaspard S, MacDougall J, Armstrong AW. Strategies to maximize clinical efficiency while maintaining patient safety during the COVID-19 pandemic: an interview-based study from private practice dermatologists. J Dermatol Treat. 2020.
6. Zarbafian M, Guo D, Dover JS, Humphrey S. The impact of COVD-19 on North American dermatology practices. J Cosmet Dermatol. 2021.
7. Cartron AM, Rismiller K, Trinidad J. Store-and-forward teledermatology in the era Of COVID-19: a pilot study. Dermatol Ther. 2020.
8. Rismiller K, Cartron AM, Trinidad J. Inpatient teledermatology during the COVID-19 pandemic. J Dermatol Treat. 2020.
9. Shourick J, Laurent C, Mion G, Skayem C, Hamann P. Impact of SARS-CoV-2 pandemic on dermatology residents: a nationwide french study. Indian J Dermatol Venereol Leprol. 2021.
10. Gehret NL, Brooks BE, Vance TM, Wambier CG, Libby TJ. Impact of the COVID-19 pandemic on dermatology residency education in the United States: a cross-sectional survey. Jaad Int. 2022.
11. Desai S, Manjaly P, Lee KJ, Li SJ, Manjaly C, Mostaghimi A. The impact of COVID-19 on dermatology clinical trials. J Invest Dermatol. 2021.
12. Weir S, Hattaway R, Singh NP, Boyd CJ, Hemal K. Characterizing the effect of the COVID-19 pandemic on the dermatology literature. Skin J Cutan Med. 2021.
13. Dréno B. What is new in the pathophysiology of acne, an overview. J Eur Acad Dermatol Venereol. 2017;31(S5):8–12.
14. Verma NK, Singh AK, Maurya AK, Rai A, Chaurasiya AK. A brief review on acne vulgaris: chronic inflammatory disease. Middle East Res J Pharm Sci. 2023;3(1):5–10.
15. Khamdan F, Shah M, Khamdan MA, Albasri EE. Acromegaly presenting with resistant acne vulgaris. Case Rep Dermatol. 2022;14(2):151–6.
16. Borzyszkowska D, Niedzielska M, Kozłowski M, Brodowska A, Przepiera A, Malczyk-Matysiak K, et al. Evaluation of hormonal factors in acne vulgaris and the course of acne vulgaris treatment with contraceptive-based therapies in young adult women. Cells. 2022;11(24):4078.
17. Albertus Alarik L, Indiastuti DN, Astari L, Setyaningrum T. The effects of hormonal factor on the degree of acne vulgaris severity. Berk Ilmu Kesehat Kulit Dan Kelamin. 2023;35(2):126–9.
18. Ryu S, Han HM, Song PI, Armstrong CA, Park Y. Suppression of propionibacterium acnes infection and the associated inflammatory response by the antimicrobial peptide P5 in mice. Picardo M, editor. PLOS ONE. 2015;10(7):e0132619.
19. Kim BS, Inan S, Ständer S, Sciascia T, Szepietowski JC, Yosipovitch G. Role of kappa-opioid and mu-opioid receptors in pruritus: peripheral and central itch circuits. Exp Dermatol. 2022;31(12):1900–7.
20. Xia X, Li Z, Liu K, Wu Y, Jiang D, Lai Y. Staphylococcal LTA-induced miR-143 inhibits propionibacterium acnes-mediated inflammatory response in skin. J Invest Dermatol. 2016;136(3):621–30.
21. Sardana K, Verma G. Propionibacterium acnes and the Th1/Th17 axis, implications … Indian J Dermatol. [cited 2024 Oct 1]. Available from: https://journals.lww.com/ijd/fulltext/2017/62040/propionibacterium_acnes_and_the_th1_th17_axis,.10.aspx
22. Carlavan I, Bertino B, Rivier M, Martel P, Bourdès V, Déret S, et al. Atrophic scar formation in patients with acne involves long-acting immune responses with plasma cells and alteration of sebaceous glands. Br J Dermatol. 2018;179(4):906–17.
23. Heng AHS, Say Y, Sio YY, Ng YT, Chew FT. Gene variants associated with acne vulgaris presentation and severity: a systematic review and meta-analysis. BMC Med Genomics. 2021;14(1).
24. Munichandrappa P, Manjunath KG, Kiran C, Variyar A. A comparative study of insulin resistance in acne vulgaris. Int J Res Dermatol. 2017;3(3):403.
25. Akpinar Kara Y, Ozdemir D. Evaluation of food consumption in patients with acne vulgaris and its relationship with acne severity. J Cosmet Dermatol. 2020;19(8):2109–13.
26. Wisuthsarewong W, Nitiyarom R, Kanchanapenkul D, Arunkajohnask S, Limphoka P, Boonchai W. Acne beliefs, treatment-seeking behaviors, information media usage, and impact on daily living activities of thai acne patients. J Cosmet Dermatol. 2019;19(5):1191–5.
27. Mahumud RA, Kamara JK, Renzaho AMN. The epidemiological burden and overall distribution of chronic comorbidities in coronavirus disease-2019 among 202,005 infected patients: evidence from

a systematic review and meta-analysis. Infection. 2020;48(6):813–33.
28. Zhang C, Shen L, Le KJ, Pan MM, Kong LC, Gu ZC, et al. Frontiers | Incidence of venous thromboembolism in hospitalized coronavirus disease 2019 patients: a systematic review and meta-analysis. [cited 2024 Oct 1]. Available from: https://www.frontiersin.org/journals/cardiovascular-medicine/articles/10.3389/fcvm.2020.00151/full
29. Cheung KS, Hung IFN, Chan PPY, Lung KC, Tso E, Liu R, et al. Gastrointestinal manifestations of SARS-CoV-2 infection and virus load in fecal samples from a Hong Kong Cohort: systematic review and meta-analysis. [cited 2024 Oct 1]. Available from: https://www.gastrojournal.org/article/S0016-5085(20)30448-0/fulltext
30. Kubota T, Kuroda N. Exacerbation of neurological symptoms and COVID-19 severity in patients with preexisting neurological disorders and COVID-19: a systematic review. Clin Neurol Neurosurg. 2021;200:106349.
31. Aziz M, Perisetti A, Lee-Smith WM, Gajendran M, Bansal P, Goyal H. Taste changes (Dysgeusia) in COVID-19: a systematic review and meta-analysis. [cited 2024 Oct 1]. Available from: https://www.gastrojournal.org/article/S0016-5085(20)30595-3/fulltext
32. Shang L, Shao M, Guo Q, Shi J, Zhao Y, Xiaokereti J, et al. Diabetes mellitus is associated with severe infection and mortality in patients with COVID-19: a systematic review and meta-analysis. Arch Med Res. 2020;51(7):700–9.
33. Sachdeva M, Mufti A, Maliyar K, Lytvyn Y, Yeung J. Hydroxychloroquine effects on psoriasis: a systematic review and a cautionary note for COVID-19 treatment. [cited 2024 Oct 1]. Available from: https://www.jaad.org/article/S0190-9622(20)30942-7/fulltext
34. Santoso A, Pranata R, Wibowo A, Al-Farabi MJ, Huang I, Antariksa B. Cardiac injury is associated with mortality and critically ill pneumonia in COVID-19: a meta-analysis. Am J Emerg Med. 2021;44:352–7.
35. Mai V, Tan BK, Mainbourg S, Potus F, Cucherat M, Lega JC, et al. Venous thromboembolism in COVID-19 compared to non-COVID-19 cohorts: a systematic review with meta-analysis. Vasc Pharmacol. 2021;139:106882.
36. Mutiawati E, Syahrul S, Fahriani M, Fajar JK, Mamada SS, Maliga HA, et al. Global prevalence and pathogenesis of headache in COVID-19: a systematic review and meta-analysis [Internet]. F1000Research;2021;9:1316 [cited 2024 Oct 1]. Available from: https://f1000research.com/articles/9-1316/v2
37. Wu X, Xu Y, Jin L, Wang X, Zhu H, Xie Y. Frontiers | Association of preexisting asthma and other allergic diseases with mortality in COVID-19 patients: a systematic review and meta-analysis. [cited 2024 Oct 1]. Available from: https://www.frontiersin.org/journals/medicine/articles/10.3389/fmed.2021.670744/full
38. Soraya GV, Ulhaq ZS. Crucial laboratory parameters in COVID-19 diagnosis and prognosis: an updated meta-analysis. Med Clínica. 2020;155(4):143–51.
39. Yousefifard M, Zali A, Zarghi A, Madani Neishaboori A, Hosseini M, Safari S. Non-steroidal anti-inflammatory drugs in management of COVID-19; a systematic review on current evidence. Int J Clin Pract. 2020;74(9):e13557.
40. Pardhan S, Wood S, Vaughan M, Trott M. Frontiers | The risk of COVID-19 related hospitalization, intensive care unit admission and mortality in people with underlying asthma or COPD: a systematic review and meta-analysis. [cited 2024 Oct 1]. Available from: https://www.frontiersin.org/journals/medicine/articles/10.3389/fmed.2021.668808/full
41. Thakur B, Dubey P, Benitez J, Torres JP, Reddy S, Shokar N, et al. A systematic review and meta-analysis of geographic differences in comorbidities and associated severity and mortality among individuals with COVID-19. Sci Rep. 2021;11(1):8562.
42. Bajgain KT, Badal S, Bajgain BB, Santana MJ. Prevalence of comorbidities among individuals with COVID-19: a rapid review of current literature. Am J Infect Control. 2021;49(2):238–46.
43. Chakraborty T, Jamal RF, Battineni G, Teja KV, Marto CM, Spagnuolo G. A review of prolonged post-COVID-19 symptoms and their implications on dental management. Int J Environ Res Public Health. 2021;18(10):5131.
44. Wang Y, Fang R, Zhang H, Tang K, Sun Q. Contributions of dermatologists to COVID-19 research: a brief systematic review. Dermatol Ther. 2020;33(4):e13713.
45. Wu L, Yuan Q, Kuang Y, Chen Y, Li J, Feng Y, et al. External treatment of traditional Chinese medicine for COVID-19: a protocol for systematic review and meta-analysis. [cited 2024 Oct 1]. Available from: https://journals.lww.com/md-journal/fulltext/2020/09250/external_treatment_of_traditional_chinese_medicine.40.aspx
46. Zhang Y, Ma P, Zhang X, Pei Z, Wang H, Dou X. Association of digestive symptoms with severity and mortality of COVID-19: a protocol for systematic review and meta-analysis. [cited 2024 Oct 1]. Available from: https://journals.lww.com/md-journal/fulltext/2020/10230/association_of_digestive_symptoms_with_severity.49.aspx
47. Ng WH, Tipih T, Makoah NA, Vermeulen JG, Goedhals D, Sempa JB, et al. Comorbidities in SARS-CoV-2 patients: a systematic review and meta-analysis. mBio. 2021;12(1). https://doi.org/10.1128/mbio.03647-20.
48. Miller MA, Cappuccio FP. A systematic review of COVID-19 and obstructive sleep apnoea. Sleep Med Rev. 2021;55:101382.
49. Fu J, Wu L, Ma Y, Liang Q. The efficacy and safety of Xuebijing injection for corona… Medicine. [cited 2024 Oct 1]; Available from: https://journals.lww.com/md-journal/fulltext/2020/12040/the_efficacy_and_safety_of_xuebijing_injection_for.64.aspx

The Effect of COVID-19 and Its Vaccination in Psoriasis Exacerbation

3

Dimitra Xenopoulou, Aleksandra Ratkiewicz, and Esraa M. AlEdani

3.1 Overview

Psoriasis is a chronic, immune-mediated, inflammatory skin disorder characterized by well-demarcated, erythematous plaques covered with silvery scales. While it predominantly affects the skin, psoriasis can also involve joints, leading to psoriatic arthritis. The prevalence of psoriasis varies, ranging from approximately 2–4% of the global population. The condition is believed to result from a complex interplay between genetic predisposition and environmental factors. At the cellular level, psoriasis is marked by the hyperproliferation of keratinocytes and the infiltration of inflammatory cells, particularly T-cells, into the skin. These mechanisms lead to accelerated skin cell turnover, resulting in the characteristic plaques of psoriasis. Due to its chronic nature, psoriasis can significantly impair quality of life, contributing to both physical discomfort and psychological distress.

Identifying and managing both triggers and exacerbating factors are critical in establishing and maintaining effective disease control. Various internal and external factors can worsen the condition, including stress, infections, trauma to the skin (Koebner phenomenon), and certain medications. Environmental factors such as cold weather, smoking, and alcohol consumption have also been implicated in the exacerbation of psoriasis. Streptococcal infections, in particular, have long been recognized as triggers for guttate psoriasis. The influence of these triggers varies among individuals, making psoriasis a highly unpredictable condition. Therefore, a comprehensive understanding of and nuanced approach to these triggers is essential for tailoring personalized treatment and management strategies to individual patients, aiming to minimize flares and improve long-term outcomes.

The COVID-19 pandemic has introduced new challenges for individuals with chronic conditions, including psoriasis. COVID-19, caused by the SARS-CoV-2 virus, is an acute respiratory illness that emerged in late 2019 and rapidly escalated into a global pandemic. The clinical manifestations of COVID-19 present with a wide spectrum of clinical manifestations from mild respiratory symptoms to severe pneumonia, acute respiratory distress syndrome (ARDS), multi-organ failure, and death. The pandemic has disrupted healthcare systems worldwide, hindering routine medical care and further complicating the management of chronic diseases like psoriasis. Moreover, the pandemic-related stress and anxiety, alongside changes in lifestyle and reduced

D. Xenopoulou · A. Ratkiewicz (✉)
New York Institute of Technology College of Osteopathic Medicine (NYITCOM), Old Westbury, NY, USA
e-mail: dxenopou@nyit.edu; aratkiew@nyit.edu

E. M. AlEdani
University of Basrah-Medical Faculty, Basrah, Iraq

E. M. AlEdani, H. Maibach (eds.), *COVID-19 Vaccination and Dermatological Diseases*, Updates in Clinical Dermatology, https://doi.org/10.1007/978-3-031-87791-9_3

access to healthcare, may have contributed to psoriasis exacerbations in affected individuals [1].

The rapid development and distribution of COVID-19 vaccines have been vital in curbing the virus' spread and reducing the severity of the disease. Several vaccines, including mRNA-based vaccines (Pfizer-BioNTech and Moderna), adenovirus vector vaccines (AstraZeneca and Johnson & Johnson), and inactivated virus vaccines (Sinopharm and Sinovac), have been authorized for emergency use globally. While these vaccines have demonstrated high efficacy in preventing COVID-19 and its severe outcomes, they have also raised concerns regarding their potential effects on individuals with chronic inflammatory conditions, such as psoriasis. Both infection and vaccination stimulate the immune system, raising questions about their potential to exacerbate autoimmune or inflammatory conditions.

The interplay between COVID-19 infection, vaccination, and psoriasis is complex and still being explored. Some studies indicate that COVID-19 infection may trigger psoriasis flares, likely due to the heightened inflammatory response induced by the virus. There are also emerging, though rare, reports of psoriasis exacerbations following COVID-19 vaccination. A better understanding of the interplay between COVID-19, its vaccination, and psoriasis is essential for developing guidelines to manage patients effectively during the ongoing pandemic and in future similar scenarios.

This paper aims to explore the effects of COVID-19 infection and its vaccination on psoriasis, providing an in-depth analysis of the current evidence and offering clinical recommendations for managing psoriasis in the context of the pandemic [2].

3.2 Impact of COVID-19 on Psoriasis Patients

The COVID-19 pandemic has posed unique challenges for individuals with chronic conditions like psoriasis. As an immune-mediated disease characterized by T-cell dysregulation, psoriasis raises concerns about how COVID-19 might affect its progression. Both the psychological stress of the pandemic and the direct effects of SARS-CoV-2 on the immune system could exacerbate psoriasis in affected individuals.

Psychological stress is a well-established trigger for psoriasis exacerbations. The pandemic has undoubtedly heightened stress levels globally due to fears of infection, social isolation, and economic uncertainties. This increase in stress has the potential to worsen psoriasis, thus leading to more frequent or severe flares. A study conducted during the early stages of the pandemic found that a significant proportion of psoriasis patients experienced exacerbations, which were attributed to heightened stress levels and lifestyle changes.

Moreover, the direct impact of COVID-19 on psoriasis patients is an area of ongoing research. Some evidence suggests that the hyperinflammatory response observed in severe COVID-19 cases may exacerbate psoriasis, which is already characterized by excessive inflammation. The cytokine storm associated with severe COVID-19, involving elevated levels of pro-inflammatory cytokines such as IL-6, TNF-α, and IL-17, mirrors the inflammatory profile of psoriasis, potentially leading to worsening of skin symptoms in infected individuals [3].

Another significant factor during the pandemic has been the disruption of routine healthcare services. Many patients with chronic conditions, including psoriasis, have faced difficulties in accessing healthcare services due to lockdowns, fear of exposure to the virus, and the reallocation of healthcare resources to manage COVID-19 patients. This disruption led to delays in follow-up appointments, interruptions of ongoing treatments, and challenges in obtaining medications, all of which may contribute to disease exacerbation.

Furthermore, the pandemic has also raised concerns about the use of systemic immunosuppressive therapies for psoriasis. Treatments such as biologics and systemic immunosuppressants, commonly prescribed in the management of moderate to severe psoriasis, could theoretically increase the risk of severe COVID-19 due to their effects on the immune system. However, current evidence suggests that the continuation of these therapies during the pandemic may not necessarily increase the risk of severe COVID-19, though this remains a topic of debate and further research.

In summary, the COVID-19 pandemic has had a multifaceted impact on individuals with psoriasis. A combination of psychological stress, potential direct effects of SARS-CoV-2, disruption of healthcare services, and concerns regarding immunosuppressive treatments have likely contributed to an increase in disease exacerbations during this time. Ongoing research is crucial to understand these interactions better and to develop clear guidelines for managing psoriasis in the context of COVID-19 [4].

3.3 Effects of COVID-19 Vaccination on Psoriasis

The rapid development and deployment of COVID-19 vaccines have been vital in controlling the spread of SARS-CoV-2. However, concerns have emerged regarding the potential effects of these vaccines on individuals with chronic inflammatory diseases like psoriasis. Since vaccines work by stimulating the immune system, there is theoretical apprehension that they could exacerbate autoimmune or inflammatory conditions.

COVID-19 vaccines- including mRNA vaccines (Pfizer-BioNTech and Moderna), adenovirus vector vaccines (AstraZeneca and Johnson & Johnson), and inactivated virus vaccines (Sinopharm and Sinovac)- have been widely administered globally. While these vaccines have shown high efficacy in preventing COVID-19 and its severe outcomes, post-marketing surveillance has revealed rare adverse events, including reports of psoriasis exacerbation following vaccination.

Emerging data suggest that most psoriasis patients tolerate COVID-19 vaccines well; however, a small subset may experience disease flares after vaccination. A review of cases reported to pharmacovigilance databases indicates that while psoriasis exacerbations post-vaccination are rare, they are noteworthy, with the majority being mild to moderate and manageable with standard psoriasis treatments. The exact mechanisms underlying these exacerbations remain unclear, but may involve immune system activation leading to an increase in pro-inflammatory cytokines, similar to those involved in psoriasis pathogenesis.

Interestingly, a study examining the safety and efficacy of the Pfizer-BioNTech vaccine in patients with autoimmune inflammatory rheumatic diseases, including psoriasis, found that the vaccine was generally well-tolerated. The study highlighted that the benefits of vaccination in preventing severe COVID-19 far outweighed the risks of potential disease exacerbation and emphasized the importance of continued monitoring and individualized care for patients with psoriasis receiving the vaccine.

In contrast, some reports suggest that COVID-19 vaccination might have a neutral or even beneficial effect on psoriasis. A subset of patients have reported stabilization or improvement of their psoriasis symptoms following vaccination, though these reports are anecdotal and require further investigation. This variability in response highlights the complexity of the immune system's interaction with vaccines and autoimmune conditions.

Given these insights, the prevailing consensus among dermatologists and rheumatologists is that COVID-19 vaccination should not be withheld from patients with psoriasis. The risk of severe COVID-19, especially in patients on immunosuppressive therapies, outweighs the potential risk of psoriasis exacerbation. However, patients with a history of severe psoriasis flares or those currently experiencing a flare are encouraged to consult with their healthcare provider before vaccination to assess the best approach.

In conclusion, while there is a small risk of psoriasis exacerbation following COVID-19 vaccination, the overall benefits of vaccination in preventing COVID-19 far exceed these risks. Ongoing monitoring and research are essential to deepen our understanding of the effects of COVID-19 vaccines on psoriasis and to inform clinical practice in this area [5].

3.4 Clinical Management of Psoriasis During the COVID-19 Pandemic

The COVID-19 pandemic has necessitated significant adjustments in the clinical management of psoriasis, a chronic condition requiring long-term treatment and regular follow-up. The challenges posed by the pandemic- including the risk of SARS-CoV-2 infection, disruptions in healthcare services, and the introduction of COVID-19 vaccines- have required dermatologists to adapt their management strategies to ensure continuity of care while minimizing risks for patients [6].

A primary concern during the pandemic has been the continuation of systemic therapies, particularly immunosuppressive treatments such as biologics and methotrexate, which are commonly used in moderate to severe psoriasis. Initially, there was uncertainty about whether these treatments could increase the risk of severe COVID-19 by suppressing the immune response. However, emerging evidence indicates that most patients can safely continue their systemic therapies with appropriate monitoring. Interrupting treatment can lead to disease flares, which pose additional risks to patients' overall health and quality of life.

Telemedicine has become an invaluable tool in the management of psoriasis during the pandemic. The use of teledermatology has facilitated remote consultations, reducing the need for in-person visits and minimizing the risk of SARS-CoV-2 exposure for both patients and healthcare providers. This approach has been particularly beneficial for patients with stable psoriasis who require regular follow-ups and prescription refills, but do not necessarily need in-person physical examinations. Moreover, many teledermatology platforms include tools for patients to upload photographs of their skin, enabling dermatologists to effectively monitor disease progression and treatment responses [7].

For patients who require in-person care- such as those undergoing phototherapy or those with severe psoriasis flares- clinics have implemented stringent infection control measures to reduce the risk of COVID-19 transmission. These measures include symptom screening, social distancing, and enhanced sanitization protocols. In some cases, the frequency of in-person visits has been reduced, and treatment regimens have been adjusted to allow for longer intervals between patient appointments.

Another significant consideration during the pandemic has been the management of psoriasis in patients who contract COVID-19. Treatment plans for these patients often need to be adjusted based on the severity of their COVID-19 symptoms and their overall health. For patients with mild, it may be possible to continue their treatments with close monitoring. Conversely, those with severe COVID-19 may require temporary discontinuation of their immunosuppressive therapies until recovery. Decisions regarding treatment adjustments should be made on a case-by-case basis, carefully weighing the risks and benefits of continuing or pausing therapy.

Vaccination has introduced further complexity into psoriasis management during the pandemic. Dermatologists must consider the timing of COVID-19 vaccination in relation to their patients' psoriasis treatments, particularly for those on immunosuppressive therapies. Some guidelines recommend temporarily holding certain treatments, such as methotrexate, around the time of vaccination to enhance vaccine efficacy, although this strategy should be individualized based on the patient's disease severity and risk of COVID-19 [8].

In conclusion, the clinical management of psoriasis during the COVID-19 pandemic requires a flexible, patient-centered approach. Ensuring continuity of care is essential, and the use of telemedicine, careful adjustment of treatment regimens, and consideration of vaccination strategies are key components of effective management. Ongoing research and updated clinical guidelines will continue to inform best practices in this challenging and evolving landscape [9].

3.5 The Role of COVID-19 Vaccinations in Psoriasis

COVID-19 vaccinations have led to varied responses in psoriasis patients, with some experiencing exacerbations while others report improvements in their symptoms. Clinical trials and observational studies examine the safety and efficacy of vaccines in this population, emphasizing the need for tailored treatment approaches [10].

During the pandemic, dermatologists have adapted management strategies by utilizing telemedicine for ongoing care and reinforcing public health guidelines. This includes educating patients on the potential effects of vaccination on their psoriasis and ensuring they receive appropriate dermatological support. Understanding the relationship between COVID-19 vaccinations and psoriasis management is essential for optimizing patient outcomes [11].

3.5.1 Review of Vaccine Types and Mechanisms

COVID-19 vaccinations have played a critical role in controlling the global pandemic, with several types developed, including mRNA vaccines (e.g., Pfizer-BioNTech and Moderna), adenovirus vector vaccines (e.g., AstraZeneca and Johnson & Johnson), and inactivated virus vaccines (e.g., Sinovac and Sinopharm). These vaccines work by stimulating the immune system to recognize and combat the SARS-CoV-2 virus.

mRNA vaccines utilize messenger RNA to instruct cells to produce a protein that triggers an immune response. In contrast, adenovirus vector vaccines employ a modified virus to deliver DNA encoding the SARS-CoV-2 spike protein. Inactivated virus vaccines contain virus particles that have been killed, effectively prompting immunity without causing disease [12].

3.5.2 Reported Cases of Psoriasis Exacerbations or Improvements Following COVID-19 Vaccination

Post-marketing surveillance and case reports have documented rare instances of psoriasis exacerbation following COVID-19 vaccination, raising interest in the vaccine's effects on autoimmune conditions like psoriasis. Some patients have reported flare-ups of psoriasis symptoms, particularly after receiving the second dose of mRNA vaccines. Generally, these flares are mild to moderate and respond well to standard psoriasis treatments. Interestingly, there are also reports of psoriasis improvement following vaccination, although such cases are less common and primarily anecdotal. This variability underscores the complex interaction between the immune system's response to vaccination and the underlying pathophysiology of psoriasis [13].

3.5.3 Clinical Trials and Observational Studies

Several studies have aimed to clarify the relationship between COVID-19 vaccination and psoriasis outcomes. Observational studies, particularly those utilizing large pharmacovigilance databases, have provided valuable insights into the safety profile of COVID-19 vaccines for psoriasis patients. While clinical trials specifically targeting this population are less common, they generally indicate that COVID-19 vaccines are safe for individuals with psoriasis, with only a small percentage experiencing disease exacerbation. Crucially, these studies highlight that the overall benefits of vaccination in preventing severe COVID-19 significantly outweigh the potential risks of psoriasis flare-ups. Ongoing research, including long-term follow-up studies, is vital for deepening our understanding of these interactions and refining vaccination guidelines for psoriasis patients [14].

3.6 Management Strategies for Psoriasis During the Pandemic

The management of psoriasis during the COVID-19 pandemic has increasingly relied on telemedicine and remote monitoring, allowing for safe consultations and ongoing care. Treatment plans have been modified to address individual patient responses to vaccination and evolving care needs. Additionally, providing psychological support has become essential in helping patients cope with increased stress and anxiety. Together, these strategies ensure optimal psoriasis management while prioritizing patient safety and well-being [15].

3.6.1 Importance of Telemedicine and Remote Monitoring

The COVID-19 pandemic has significantly accelerated the adoption of telemedicine, transforming it into a vital tool for managing chronic conditions like psoriasis. Teledermatology enables remote consultations, allowing patients to receive care without the need for in-person visits and thereby reducing the risk of SARS-CoV-2 exposure. Many telemedicine platforms offer features that permit patients to upload images of their skin, facilitating real-time assessments by dermatologists. This capability has proven especially valuable for monitoring disease progression, adjusting treatment plans, and ensuring continuity of care during the pandemic [16].

3.6.2 Modification of Treatment Plans

The pandemic has necessitated modifications to treatment plans for psoriasis patients, especially those receiving immunosuppressive therapies. Initially, there were concerns that these treatments could heighten the risk of severe COVID-19. However, emerging evidence indicates that many patients can safely continue these therapies with appropriate monitoring. Treatment adjustments, such as switching to less immunosuppressive agents or spacing out doses, have been implemented on a case-by-case basis to balance effective disease control with the potential risk of COVID-19 complications. Furthermore, the rollout of COVID-19 vaccinations has required careful timing of immunosuppressive treatments to maximize vaccine efficacy while minimizing the risk of psoriasis exacerbation [17].

3.6.3 Psychological Support for Patients

The psychological impact of the pandemic, characterized by heightened stress and anxiety, has been particularly profound for individuals with chronic conditions like psoriasis, which is known to worsen under stress. Providing psychological support to psoriasis patients during this challenging time is essential. This support may encompass counseling, stress management strategies, and access to mental health resources. Integrating psychological care into psoriasis management plans can help alleviate the effects of pandemic-related stress on disease outcomes [18].

3.7 Considerations for Psoriasis Patients Regarding COVID-19 Vaccination

When it comes to COVID-19 vaccination, psoriasis patients must be informed about the safety and efficacy of available vaccines, particularly regarding their specific health conditions and treatments. Healthcare providers should counsel patients on the benefits of vaccination, such as reducing the risk of severe illness, while also addressing potential risks, including any concerns about exacerbations of their condition. Additionally, it is crucial to engage with patients experiencing vaccine hesitancy, providing clear, evidence-based information to alleviate fears and encourage informed decision-making. This comprehensive approach empowers psoriasis patients to make confident choices about their health during the pandemic [19].

3.7.1 Safety and Efficacy of COVID-19 Vaccines in Psoriasis Patients

COVID-19 vaccines have been found to be generally safe and effective for patients with psoriasis, with most studies indicating that the benefits of vaccination significantly outweigh the associated risks. Although there are some reports of psoriasis exacerbations following vaccination, these instances are rare, and the majority of patients do not experience significant adverse effects. Crucially, vaccination greatly reduces the risk of severe COVID-19, which can have serious consequences, particularly for individuals with underlying health conditions. For psoriasis patients undergoing systemic immunosuppressive therapies, careful management of the vaccination timing in relation to their treatment schedule may be necessary to optimize the vaccine's effectiveness [20].

3.7.2 Counseling Patients on Benefits and Risks

Counseling psoriasis patients about the benefits and risks of COVID-19 vaccination is crucial. Healthcare providers should offer clear and balanced information, highlighting that while there is a small risk of psoriasis flares, the vaccine's protection against severe COVID-19 is vital. Patients should be informed about the potential for mild side effects, including possible exacerbations of psoriasis, and reassured that these can typically be managed effectively with appropriate treatment. Developing individualized care plans that consider the patient's disease severity, treatment regimen, and overall health is essential for facilitating informed decision-making regarding vaccination [21].

3.7.3 Addressing Vaccine Hesitancy

Vaccine hesitancy among some psoriasis patients, particularly those concerned about potential disease flares, is a significant issue. To address this hesitancy, it is essential to provide evidence-based information regarding the safety of COVID-19 vaccines for psoriasis patients, while also discussing the risks of remaining unvaccinated, including the potential for severe COVID-19. Healthcare providers should foster open and empathetic communication, addressing specific concerns and misconceptions, and emphasizing the importance of vaccination as a vital tool for maintaining health during the pandemic. By ensuring that patients feel supported and well-informed, providers can help alleviate vaccine-related anxiety and promote higher vaccination rates [22].

3.8 Conclusion

The COVID-19 pandemic has posed unique and significant challenges in the management of psoriasis, a chronic inflammatory condition characterized by complex interactions between the immune system and environmental factors. This paper examines the multifaceted effects of COVID-19 and its vaccinations on psoriasis, emphasizing the role of immune mechanisms, patient management strategies, and the critical importance of vaccination. While evidence indicates a risk of psoriasis exacerbation following COVID-19 vaccination, these risks are generally outweighed by the benefits, particularly in preventing severe COVID-19. Moreover, the pandemic has also underscored the value of telemedicine in establishing and maintaining continuity of care, facilitating remote monitoring, and minimizing the risk of infection.

Effective management of psoriasis during the pandemic requires a flexible, patient-centered approach. Key adjustments to treatment plans, such as modifying immunosuppressive regimens and incorporating psychological support, have been essential in maintaining disease control and enhancing patient well-being. Current evidence supports the safety and efficacy of COVID-19 vaccinations in psoriasis patients, highlighting the need for ongoing monitoring and individualized care.

Looking ahead, the lessons learned from managing psoriasis during the pandemic will have enduring implications for clinical practice. The integration of telemedicine into routine care, the importance of psychological support, and the careful management of immunosuppressive therapies in the context of vaccination are likely to continue influencing psoriasis management strategies. Furthermore, ongoing research is essential to further elucidate the long-term effects of COVID-19 and its vaccines on psoriasis, ultimately refining both treatment and vaccination guidelines.

In conclusion, the intersection of psoriasis and COVID-19 presents both challenges and opportunities for advancing patient care. The pandemic has reinforced the importance of adaptable, patient-focused care and the need for continued research to ensure optimal outcomes for psoriasis patients in an evolving healthcare landscape.

References

1. Agarwal A, Panda M, Behera BK, Jena AK. Benign cutaneous reactions post-COVID-19 vaccination: a case series of 16 patients from a tertiary care center in India. J Cosmet Dermatol. 2022;21(1):30–3. https://doi.org/10.1111/jocd.14592.
2. Aryanian Z, Balighi K, Hatami P, Goodarzi A, Mohandesi NA, Afshar ZM. SARS-CoV-2 vaccination and practical points in psoriasis patients: a narrative review. Dermatol Ther. 2022;35(5). https://doi.org/10.1111/dth.15430.
3. Campanati A, Diotallevi F, Martina E, Radi G, Offidani A. Treatment of moderate to severe psoriasis during the COVID-19 pandemic: lessons learned and opportunities. J Clin Med. 2022;11(9):2422. https://doi.org/10.3390/jcm11092422.
4. Gambichler T, Boms S, Susok L, et al. Cutaneous findings following COVID-19 vaccination: review of world literature and own experience. J Eur Acad Dermatol Venereol. 2022;36(2):172–80. https://doi.org/10.1111/jdv.17744.
5. Heil M. Self-DNA driven inflammation in COVID-19 and after mRNA-based vaccination: lessons for non-COVID-19 pathologies. Front Immunol. 2024;14:1259879. https://doi.org/10.3389/fimmu.2023.1259879.
6. Huang YW, Tsai TF. Exacerbation of psoriasis following COVID-19 vaccination: report from a single center. Front Med (Lausanne). 2021;8:812010. https://doi.org/10.3389/fmed.2021.812010.
7. Karampinis E, Papadopoulou MM, Chaidaki K, et al. Plaque psoriasis exacerbation and COVID-19 vaccination: assessing the characteristics of the flare and the exposome parameters. Vaccines (Basel). 2024;12(2):178. https://doi.org/10.3390/vaccines12020178.
8. Khandker SS, Godman B, Jawad MI, et al. A systematic review on COVID-19 vaccine strategies, their effectiveness, and issues. Vaccines (Basel). 2021;9(12):1387. https://doi.org/10.3390/vaccines9121387.
9. Kocivnik N, Velnar T. A review pertaining to SARS-CoV-2 and autoimmune diseases: what is the connection? Life (Basel). 2022;12(11):1918. https://doi.org/10.3390/life12111918.
10. Lodde GC, Krefting F, Placke JM, et al. COVID-19 vaccination in psoriasis patients receiving systemic treatment: a prospective single-center study. Front Immunol. 2023;14:1107438. https://doi.org/10.3389/fimmu.2023.1107438.
11. Martora F, Battista T, Ruggiero A, et al. The impact of COVID-19 vaccination on inflammatory skin disorders and other cutaneous diseases: a review of the published literature. Viruses. 2023;15(7):1423. https://doi.org/10.3390/v15071423.
12. Musumeci ML, Caruso G, Trecarichi AC, Micali G. Safety of SARS-CoV-2 vaccines in psoriatic patients treated with biologics: a real-life experience. Dermatol Ther. 2022;35(1). https://doi.org/10.1111/dth.15177.
13. Niebel D, Novak N, Wilhelmi J, et al. Cutaneous adverse reactions to COVID-19 vaccines: insights from an immuno-dermatological perspective. Vaccines (Basel). 2021;9(9):944. https://doi.org/10.3390/vaccines9090944.
14. Piaserico S, Gisondi P, Cazzaniga S, Di Leo S, Naldi L. Assessing the risk and outcome of COVID-19 in patients with psoriasis or psoriatic arthritis on biologic treatment: a critical appraisal of the quality of the published evidence. J Invest Dermatol. 2022;142(2):355–63.e7. https://doi.org/10.1016/j.jid.2021.04.036.
15. Polack FP, Thomas SJ, Kitchin N, et al. Safety and efficacy of the BNT162b2 mRNA Covid-19 vaccine. N Engl J Med. 2020;383(27):2603–15. https://doi.org/10.1056/NEJMoa2034577.
16. Potestio L, Martora F, Fabbrocini G, Battista T, Megna M. Safety and efficacy of Covid-19 vaccination in patients undergoing biological treatments for psoriasis. Psoriasis (Auckl). 2023;13:11–8. https://doi.org/10.2147/PTT.S398135.
17. Shah H, Busquets AC. Psoriasis flares in patients with COVID-19 infection or vaccination: a case series. Cureus. 2022;14(6). https://doi.org/10.7759/cureus.25987.
18. Sotiriou E, Tsentemeidou A, Bakirtzi K, Lallas A, Ioannides D, Vakirlis E. Psoriasis exacerbation after COVID-19 vaccination: a report of 14 cases from a single centre. J Eur Acad Dermatol Venereol. 2021;35(12). https://doi.org/10.1111/jdv.17582.
19. Voysey M, Clemens SAC, Madhi SA, et al. Safety and efficacy of the ChAdOx1 nCoV-19 vaccine (AZD1222) against SARS-CoV-2: an interim analysis of four randomised controlled trials in Brazil, South Africa, and the UK. Lancet. 2021;397(10269):99–111. https://doi.org/10.1016/S0140-6736(20)32661-1.
20. Weschawalit S, Pongcharoen P, Suthiwartnarueput W, et al. Cutaneous adverse events after COVID-19

vaccination. Clin Cosmet Investig Dermatol. 2023;16:1473–84. https://doi.org/10.2147/CCID.S410690.

21. Wu PC, Huang IH, Wang CW, Tsai CC, Chung WH, Chen CB. New onset and exacerbations of psoriasis following COVID-19 vaccines: a systematic review. Am J Clin Dermatol. 2022;23(6):775–99. https://doi.org/10.1007/s40257-022-00721-z.

22. Mroz M, Mućka S, Miodońska M, Ziolkowska D, Hadas E, Bożek A. Influence of SARS-CoV-2 virus infection on the course of psoriasis during treatment with biological drugs. Medicina (Kaunas). 2021;57(9):881. https://doi.org/10.3390/medicina57090881.

Impact of COVID-19 and Its Vaccination on Cutaneous Lupus Erythematosus

4

Nereen A. Almosilhy and Esraa M. AlEdani

Abbreviations

ACLE	Acute Cutaneous Lupus Erythematosus
ANAs	Antinuclear Antibodies
CCLE	Chronic Cutaneous Lupus Erythematosus
CDLE	Chronic Discoid Lupus Erythematosus
ChLE	Chilblain Lupus Erythematosus
CLE	Cutaneous Lupus Erythematosus
ICLE	Intermittent Cutaneous Lupus Erythematosus
LE	Lupus Erythematosus
SCLE	Subacute Cutaneous Lupus Erythematosus
SLE	Systematic Lupus Erythematosus
TEN	Toxic Epidermal Necrolysis

4.1 Overview of Cutaneous Lupus Erythematosus (CLE)

Lupus erythematosus (LE) is an autoimmune disease characterized by a wide range of signs and symptoms, from cutaneous lesions to extensive systemic manifestations, as seen in systemic lupus erythematosus (SLE). Among individuals with SLE, 70–80% develop skin-related symptoms during their illness, and in 20–25% of these patients, skin lesions are the initial sign of the disease [1]. Cutaneous lupus erythematosus (CLE) can present either as an independent skin condition or as one of the manifestations associated with SLE [2]. Both SLE and CLE predominantly affect females more than males [3]. Annually, the United States and Europe report approximately 4 cases of CLE compared to 3 cases of SLE per 100,000 individuals [4, 5]. CLE is a devastating disease that significantly reduces patients' quality of life due to its persistent nature, tendency to affect exposed skin areas, and disfiguring effects [6].

N. A. Almosilhy (✉)
Department of Pharmacology and Toxicology, Faculty of Pharmacy, Tanta University, Tanta, Egypt

E. M. AlEdani
University of Basrah-Medical Faculty, Basrah, Iraq

4.2 Classification of CLE

Considering the clinical signs, histopathological features, serological markers, and disease duration, CLE-specific skin manifestations are categorized into four types:

- Acute CLE (ACLE): Represents approximately 15% of CLE cases and often presents as a localized butterfly rash symmetrically affecting the malar areas of the face or as widespread erythema in sun-exposed areas. It is closely linked to SLE often reflecting overall disease activity, with a high prevalence of specific anti-

E. M. AlEdani, H. Maibach (eds.), *COVID-19 Vaccination and Dermatological Diseases*, Updates in Clinical Dermatology, https://doi.org/10.1007/978-3-031-87791-9_4

bodies (e.g., antinuclear antibodies [ANAs], present in about 80% of cases, or anti-double-stranded DNA antibodies in 30–40%) and common systematic symptoms like fever and fatigue driven by type I interferons [5]. A rare form of ACLE, known as the TEN-like variant, mimics toxic epidermal necrolysis (TEN), which is characterized by severe interface dermatitis and the death of keratinocytes, leading to the detachment of large skin areas. While mucosal regions may be involved, the ocular conjunctiva is typically unaffected. After resolution, ACLE lesions may cause residual hyperpigmentation but rarely result in scarring, except in TEN-like variants or when complicated by a secondary infection [7].

- Subacute CLE (SCLE): Accounts for approximately 8% of CLE cases and manifests as psoriasiform papulosquamous or polycyclic annular lesions, or both, in the same patient. These lesions typically appear symmetrically on sun-exposed areas such as the neck, shoulders, arms, upper trunk, and legs, and rarely affect the face. Unlike other CLE subtypes, SCLE lesions generally do not show significant atrophy or keratosis and tend to be less edematous and dyschromic [8]. Some SCLE-reported cases are drug-induced, associated with medications like hydrochlorothiazide, angiotensin-converting enzyme inhibitors (ACEI), calcium channel blockers, proton-pump inhibitors (PPIs), terbinafine, anticonvulsants, antineoplastic agents, and anti-TNF agents [9–12]. SCLE can also be associated with malignancies, functioning as a paraneoplastic syndrome in rare instances [13].
- Intermittent CLE (ICLE): Also referred to as lupus erythematosus tumidus (LET), ICLE is characterized by alternating periods of remission and recurrence, along with extreme photosensitivity [14]. It features non-scarring, non-scaling lesions on sun-exposed skin and can occasionally coexist with other CLE forms, such as discoid lupus erythematosus (DLE), but rarely with SLE. Its classification remains debated and may be considered a subtype of chronic CLE (CCLE) [15].
- Chronic CLE (CCLE): Represents over 70% of all CLE cases and is characterized by a long-lasting, gradually progressing course with variable systemic associations [16]. It includes several subtypes, the most common of which is chronic discoid lupus erythematosus (CDLE), comprising approximately 50% of CCLE cases and present in about 20% of SLE patients. CDLE manifests as scarring plaques with adherent scales, typically in a discoid shape. Lesions can be localized to areas such as the face, neck, and scalp or disseminated (spreading more widely across the body). CCLE may sometimes exhibit hyperkeratosis (hypertrophic type), leading to scarring and cicatricial alopecia when affecting hair-bearing regions [17, 18]. Anti-TNF agents and certain chemotherapeutics drugs have rarely been reported to induce DLE [19]. Rare CCLE variants include lupus erythematosus profundus, which affects the subcutaneous fat, and chilblain lupus erythematosus (ChLE), which mainly impacts acral surfaces such as the ears, nose, fingers, and toes, and it is often triggered by cold exposure. ChLE may coexist with DLE or occur in association with SLE and it is linked to Raynaud's phenomenon. Additional rare CCLE variants include comedonic lupus erythematosus, mucosal discoid lupus erythematosus, hypertrophic lupus erythematosus (Verrucous LE), and lichen planus-like lupus erythematosus.

Other rare CLE variants include bullous CLE, neonatal CLE, mucocutaneous lupus, and Rowell syndrome [20–22]. Internal organ involvement can complicate CLE, regardless of subtype. The incidence of systemic symptoms varies by CLE subtype; for example, ACLE is associated with systemic involvement in approximately 90% of cases, whereas localized CDLE shows such involvement in fewer than 5% of cases [23, 24]. CLE is also associated with other non-specific skin disorders common in autoimmune diseases, including vascular conditions and hair follicle diseases like alopecia [16, 25, 26].

4.3 Molecular Pathogenesis of CLE

The molecular pathogenesis of CLE involves a complex interplay between genetic susceptibility and key environmental factors, including UV light and cigarette smoke. These factors trigger an anti-epithelial cytotoxic immune response and create a self-amplifying proinflammatory cycle that exacerbates the disease.

CLE skin lesions are marked by the expression of type I interferon-regulated proinflammatory cytokines. Gene expression studies reveal that both innate and adaptive immune pathways are simultaneously activated in CLE lesions. Innate pathways involve proinflammatory cytokines, chemokines, complement activation, DNA/RNA recognition, and cell death. Adaptive pathways include leukocyte migration, T and B cell activation, and antigen presentation. Keratinocytes might also contribute to lesion formation by producing type I and type III interferons and proinflammatory cytokines like CXCL10, promoting immune cell recruitment and keratinocyte death through mechanisms such as necroptosis [27]. Additionally, CLE gene expression profiles significantly overlap with those observed in other autoimmune diseases, type I interferon-mediated antiviral responses, and anti-epithelial disorders [28–31].

Regarding genetic susceptibility in CLE, only one monogenic variant of CLE, a rare familial form of ChLE caused by a TREX1 mutation, has been identified to date. TREX1 deficiency leads to persistent activation of the type I interferon system through cytosolic DNA sensing pathways [32]. Beyond this, various genetic associations, including mutations and polymorphisms, have been reported in different CLE populations [33]. These genetic factors affects components of both innate and adaptive immune systems, including interferon signaling pathway, antigen presentation, antibody production, cell death, debris clearance, and immune cell regulation.

Furthermore, CLE can be induced by certain drugs, including some antihypertensives, PPIs, anticonvulsants, antineoplastic agents, TNF-blockers, and immune stimulators (e.g., checkpoint inhibitors), which activate the innate immune system either directly or indirectly or disrupt interferon regulation, resulting in increased pro-inflammatory interferon factors [34–39].

4.4 Shared Pathogenic Mechanisms Between COVID-19 and CLE

COVID-19, caused by severe acute respiratory syndrome coronavirus 2 (SARS-CoV-2), was first identified in Wuhan, China, in December 2019 and was declared a pandemic in March 2020 [40]. It has resulted in an estimated 14.83 million deaths globally, making it the most tragic health crisis since the 1918 influenza pandemic [41]. Ongoing outbreaks continue due to viral mutations that have led to multiple variants, though only a few are classified as variants of concern (VOCs).

COVID-19 progresses through acute and chronic phases, presenting with a wide range of clinical symptoms, including fever, cough, shortness of breath, and skin lesions [42, 43]. Between 1.8% and nearly 25% of COVID-19 patients develop dermatological manifestations, which may appear in various body areas [44, 45]. These cutaneous lesions along with alterations in pro-inflammatory mediators such as interferons, resemble the physiological and pathological features observed in CLE [43, 46]. Although genetic, autoimmune, molecular, environmental, and drug-related factors are recognized contributors to CLE development, the connection between COVID-19 and CLE remains underexplored. Recent reports have highlighted an growing number of cases in which individuals experience CLE flare-ups following COVID-19 infection or vaccination.

A recent interesting study by Gao et al. (2023) explored gene expression patterns to uncover common pathogenic mechanisms between COVID-19 and CLE. Through the analysis of two datasets, GSE171110 (COVID-19) and GSE109248 (CLE), the researchers identified 214 overlapping differentially expressed genes (DEGs) [47]. Functional enrichment analysis revealed that these DEGs are associated with viral responses, immune receptor activity, and double-stranded RNA binding, all of which trigger immune signaling cascade that lead to the production of type I and III interferons, which exert antiviral effects both directly and indirectly. Further analysis using KEGG pathways identified 15 significant pathways associated with the overlapping DEGs. These include pathways related to COVID-19, Influenza A, Epstein-Barr virus (EBV) infection, *Staphylococcus aureus* infection, complement and coagulation cascades, and the differentiation of Th1 and Th2 cells. Notably, the Coronavirus infectious diseases had the highest number of shared DEGs, suggesting that bacterial and viral infections may contribute to the pathogenesis of both COVID-19 and CLE. This is further supported by a case report describing the onset of pediatric SLE symptoms in a previously healthy 14-year-old girl three months after acquiring the Omicron variant of COVID-19 and EBV infections [48].

Moreover, Gao and colleagues performed a protein-protein interaction (PPI) network and identified five key hub genes (IRF7, RSAD2, IFIH1, IFIT1, IFIT3), all of which are involved in antiviral and immune responses. *IRF7 (Interferon Regulatory Factor 7) is central regulator of type I interferon–dependent antiviral immune responses and has been associated with increased COVID-19 severity, particularly among African Americans [49]. In addition, IRF7 is a key factor in CLE, marked by increased interferon responses in lupus keratinocytes [50]. *RSAD2 (radical S-adenosyl methionine domain containing 2) is an interferon-stimulated antiviral protein and is essential for the cellular response to viral infections mediated by both type I and type II interferons. Its expression has been found elevated in patients with COVID-19 and CDLE, indicating its potential as a therapeutic target [51]. *IFIH1 (interferon-induced with helicase C domain 1) is responsible for sensing viral RNA, triggering the innate immune signaling, and regulating type I interferon production during SARS-CoV-2 infections [52]. It is also involved in several inflammatory diseases, with increased expression observed in the skin of patients with CDLE and lichen planus [53]. *IFIT1 and IFIT3 (interferon-induced proteins with tetratricopeptide repeats 1 and 3), both are interferon-activated antiviral proteins that inhibit viral activities and cellular processes, including cell signaling, proliferation, migration, and the replication of viruses. The increased expression of these genes has been observed in SARS-CoV-2–infected cells, indicating the activation of the innate immune response [54].

4.5 Clinical Case Studies Linking COVID-19 Infection with CLE

Several case studies have explored the relationship between COVID-19, CLE, and SLE, ranging from new-onset presentations of rare CLE variants in previously healthy individuals to disease flare-ups in patients with established lupus diagnosis. For instance, COVID-19 triggered lupus panniculitis in a 66-year-old woman, marking her first manifestation of SLE following a COVID-19 infection [55]. In another case, a severe form of CLE resembling TEN was reported in a 70-year-old woman one month after recovering from COVID-19 [56]. A comparative study by Battesti et al. (2020) examined seven cases of COVID–19–associated chilblains (also termed epidemic chilblains or EC) and eleven cases of ChLE. COVID-19-associated chilblains were restricted to the feet, whereas ChLE lesions involved the hands, ears, or nose in 82% of cases. Autoimmune markers, like ANA, were absent in the COVID-19 group but present in 91% of ChLE cases. Both groups showed strong interferon responses but differed in histopathological features, suggesting that COVID–19–related chilblains are primarily mediated by immune dysregulation rather than direct active viral replication [57].

Furthermore, in patients with preexisting CLE, a 67-year-old woman with CCLE developed a Rowell syndrome–like flare two weeks after recovering from a mild COVID-19 infection [58]. A rare case of sudden-onset wall-eyed bilateral internuclear ophthalmoplegia (WEBINO) syndrome was reported two months after recovering from COVID-19 in a patient with SCLE, highlighting neurological complications triggered by COVID-19 infection in patients with preexisting autoimmune diseases like lupus [59]. These findings emphasize the need for close post-COVID monitoring and adherence to COVID-19 preventive practices in lupus patients.

4.6 COVID-19 Vaccination and Its Association with CLE Flare-Ups

The U.S. Food and Drug Administration (FDA) authorized the emergency use of prominent COVID-19 vaccines based on their efficacy and response to emerging variants, resulting in the global administration of 13,501,307,588 vaccine doses [60, 61]. However, multiple case reports and letters have documented the onset or exacerbation of CLE and related autoimmune conditions following COVID-19 vaccinations, including AstraZeneca, Pfizer-BioNTech, Moderna, and BBIBP-CorV. These cases involved patients with various CLE subtypes, such as SCLE, CCLE, and rare variant subtypes, and were observed in both healthy individuals and those with preexisting conditions (Table 4.1). Among the reported cases, patients experienced symptoms such as flare-ups, rashes, pruritus, burning sensations, erythema, and hypopigmentation. In some instances, existing lupus worsened or transitioned into systemic forms, while in others, new lupus-related symptoms developed following vaccination.

Notable cases include a 51-year-old man with SLE and Sjögren's syndrome who developed discoid subacute CLE after receiving AstraZeneca vaccine. His condition resolved with residual vitiligo-like post-inflammatory depigmentation. Another case involved a 24-year-old woman whose lupus symptoms worsened, accompanied by new-onset SCLE after the Pfizer-BioNTech vaccine.

Additional reports include a 30-year-old Italian woman with primary biliary cholangitis who developed SCLE, demonstrating vaccine-induced flares with some hypopigmentation remaining; and a 71-year-old man with SLE and type 2 diabetes controlled by dipeptidyl peptidase-4 inhibitors (DPP-4I) who developed both bullous SLE and dipeptidyl peptidase-4 inhibitor-associated bullous pemphigoid (DPP-4i-BP) after his COVID-19 vaccination, which was linked to both the vaccine and his DPP-4I treatment. Moreover, a 30-year-old woman in Iran developed DLE following a COVID-19 infection and subsequently experienced a flare-up after receiving her third dose of the BBIBP-CorV vaccine.

In another instance, a 62-year-old woman with SCLE developed SLE ten days after receiving the AstraZeneca vaccine. Additionally, a 54-year-old woman with SCLE experienced a flare four days after her first Moderna vaccine dose, and in Brazil, a 40-year-old woman with CCLE affecting the scalp experienced an exacerbation approximately one month after receiving her second AstraZeneca vaccine dose.

These cases suggest that while lupus flares post-vaccination are rare, they may occur, especially in predisposed individuals. Despite these incidents, the overall benefits of COVID-19 vaccination outweigh the risks. Clinicians are advised to closely monitor patients with autoimmune conditions after vaccination to ensure rapid identification and management of potential flares effectively.

Table 4.1 Reported cases of cutaneous and systemic lupus erythematosus following COVID-19 vaccination

Study ID	Country	Sex/ Age (years)	comorbidities	Type of vaccine	Dose	Duration between vaccination and symptom onset	Clinical symptoms and CLE subtype
Joseph and Chong (2021) [62]	USA	F/54	SCLE	mRNA (Moderna)	1st	4 days	Exacerbation of SCLE with increased pruritis, erythema, and burning sensation
Liu and Messenger (2021) [63]	USA	M/70	lung cancer	mRNA (Pfizer-BioNTech, BNT162b2)	2nd	10 weeks	New onset of SCLE; violaceous plaques with central depigmentation, surrounding redness, peripheral scaling on upper limbs, abdomen, and back; positive ANA
Zengarini et al. (2022) [64]	Italy	F/30	Primary biliary cholangitis	mRNA (Pfizer, Comirnaty)	2nd	10 days	SCLE-papules and erythematous plaques on face and upper back; resolved with post-inflammatory hypopigmentation on back
Niebel et al. (2021) [65]	Germany	F/73	SCLE, Raynaud's syndrome with digital ulcerations, joint pain, hair loss	mRNA (BNT162b2, Pfizer)	1st	10 days	Exacerbation of SCLE: widespread burning erythematous patches
Rechtien et al. (2022) [66]	Germany	F/24	SLE, lupus panniculitis, anemia	mRNA (BNT162b2, Pfizer)	1st and 2nd	14 days after 1st and 4 days after 2nd	New onset SCLE-solitary papular eruptions on the chest after 1st dose and pruritic papulosquamous exanthema on proximal limbs and upper trunk
Kreuter et al. (2021) [67]	Germany	F/62	SCLE	Adenoviral (AZD1222)	1st	10 days	Transition from SCLE to SLE, fatigue, and musculoskeletal pain; widespread erythematous macules
Kreuter et al. (2022) [68]	Germany	M/79	–	mRNA (BNT162b2)	1st	10 days	SCLE-annular and papulosquamous exanthema on the trunk and lower legs
Rose et al. (2022) [69]	USA	F/33	–	mRNA (BNT162b2 Pfizer)	2nd	Within hours	CLE-like reaction with vacuolar interface alteration, perivascular and periadnexal lymphocytic infiltrate
Bakr et al. (2022) [70]	UK	M/51	SLE and Sjogren's syndrome	Adenoviral (AZD1222)	1st and 2nd	7 days after 1st dose, 4 days after 2nd dose	Flat papules on hands dorsum, scalp, and ears; Discoid subacute CLE- erythematous annular polycyclic lesions on scalp, arms, trunk, and back; palmar perniosis; resolved with vitiligo-like post-inflammatory depigmentation

(continued)

Table 4.1 (continued)

Study ID	Country	Sex/ Age (years)	comorbidities	Type of vaccine	Dose	Duration between vaccination and symptom onset	Clinical symptoms and CLE subtype
Nakahara et al. (2023) [71]	Japan	M/71	SLE, HLH, and DM Type 2 controlled by DPP-4i	mRNA (Pfizer–BioNTech)	1st and 2nd	14 days after 1st dose, 40 after 2nd dose	Conversion from SLE to bullous SLE, multiple blisters on arms, and neck; DPP-4i-BP
Rimmer et al. (2023) [72]	USA	F/79	Hypothyroidism, Essential thrombocytosis	mRNA (Moderna)	2nd	14 days	SCLE-like eruption, pruritic exanthem to shoulders, breasts, chest, abdomen, and back; scalp erythema; ridged fingernails
Famularo et al. (2023) [73]	Italy	F/70	Hypertension	Adenoviral (ChAdOx1 nCoV-19)	1st	48 h	New-onset CLE with erythematous plaques on trunk, upper and lower limb; positive ANA; muscle pain, arthralgias
Souza et al. (2024) [74]	Brazil	F/40	CCLE on the scalp	Adenoviral (ChAdOx1 nCoV-19)	2nd	30 days	Exacerbation of CCLE, scalp burning itching erythema, with serohematic exudate, and alopecia with erythematous scaly papules and plaques; rough, dry lupus hair shafts
Pour Mohammad et al (2024) [75]	Iran	F/30	–	BBIBP-CorV	3rd	–	One-month post-COVID infection; DLE-itchy erythematous forehead papules; scaly scalp with focal alopecia; lesions expanded to neck and back within a week; flare-up after 3rd COVID-19 vaccination

M male, *F* female, *SLE* systematic lupus erythematosus, *CLE* cutaneous lupus erythematosus, *SCLE* subacute cutaneous lupus erythematosus, *CCLE* chronic cutaneous lupus erythematosus, *DLE* discoid lupus erythematosus, *DM* diabetes miletus, *HLH* hemophagocytic lymphohistiocytosis, *DPP-4i* dipeptidyl peptidase 4 inhibitors, *DPP-4i-BP* dipeptidyl peptidase 4 inhibitors-associated bullous pemphigoid, *ANA* antinuclear antibodies

4.7 Management Strategies for CLE During the COVID-19 Pandemic

The treatment plan for patients experiencing vaccine-induced CLE or an exacerbation of lupus conditions following COVID-19 vaccination or infection typically involves a combination of medications, regular follow-up care to monitor progress, and patient education. Patients are commonly treated with immunosuppressive and anti-inflammatory medications to manage the disease activity and control flare-ups. Commonly prescribed drugs include corticosteroids and antimalarials like hydroxychloroquine, which are effective in reducing inflammation and alleviating lupus symptoms, particularly at increased doses for those already using them for

SLE. Topical corticosteroids, such as mometasone, may also be applied to manage local inflammation. In more severe cases, systematic immunosuppressive therapies, such as azathioprine, may be necessary to suppress the immune activity and prevent further skin damage.

Furthermore, CLE patients are advised to avoid known triggers such as UV radiation and cigarette smoking, which can exacerbate the condition. Preventive measures for CLE patients, including the consistent use of sunscreen, protective clothing, and lifestyle modifications, are essential for disease management. In addition, minimizing the risk of COVID-19 infection can be achieved by practicing proper hand hygiene, using protective equipment, and maintaining social distancing.

For instance, a study from Bergamo, Italy, a high-epidemic area during the COVID-19 pandemic, discusses the implementation of strict preventive measures while continuing treatment management for CLE and SLE patients. Among 25 patients, none discontinued therapy, and lupus symptoms remained stable. Only four developed mild COVID-19 symptoms, with no hospitalizations or significant lupus flare-ups. This reflects the importance of maintaining preventive measures and the continuation of treatments during the pandemic [76].

References

1. Jarukitsopa S, Hoganson DD, Crowson CS, Sokumbi O, Davis MD, Michet CJ, et al. Epidemiology of systemic lupus erythematosus and cutaneous lupus erythematosus in a predominantly white population in the United States. Arthritis Care Res. 2015;67(6):817–28.
2. Wenzel J. Cutaneous lupus erythematosus: new insights into pathogenesis and therapeutic strategies. Nat Rev Rheumatol. 2019;15(9):519–32.
3. Vale ECSD, Garcia LC. Cutaneous lupus erythematosus: a review of etiopathogenic, clinical, diagnostic and therapeutic aspects. An Bras Dermatol. 2023;98(3):355–72.
4. Durosaro O, Davis MDP, Reed KB, Rohlinger AL. Incidence of cutaneous lupus erythematosus, 1965-2005: a population-based study. Arch Dermatol. 2009;145(3):249–53.
5. Biazar C, Sigges J, Patsinakidis N, Ruland V, Amler S, Bonsmann G, et al. Cutaneous lupus erythematosus: first multicenter database analysis of 1002 patients from the European Society of Cutaneous Lupus Erythematosus (EUSCLE). Autoimmun Rev. 2013;12(3):444–54.
6. Batalla A, García-Doval I, Peón G, de la Torre C. A quality-of-life study of cutaneous lupus erythematosus. Actas Dermosifiliogr (Engl Ed). 2013;104(9):800–6.
7. Roberts EJ, Melchionda V, Saldanha G, Shaffu S, Royle J, Harman KE. Toxic epidermal necrolysis-like lupus. Clin Exp Dermatol. 2021;46(7):1299–303.
8. Blake SC, Daniel BS. Cutaneous lupus erythematosus: a review of the literature. Int J Womens Dermatol. 2019;5(5):320–9.
9. Michaelis TC, Sontheimer RD, Lowe GC. An update in drug-induced subacute cutaneous lupus erythematosus. Dermatol Online J. 2017;23(3).
10. He Y, Sawalha AH. Drug-induced lupus erythematosus: an update on drugs and mechanisms. Curr Opin Rheumatol. 2018;30(5):490–7.
11. Borucki R, Werth VP. Cutaneous lupus erythematosus induced by drugs—novel insights. Expert Rev Clin Pharmacol. 2020;13(1):35–42.
12. Bataille P, Chasset F, Monfort JB, De Risi-Pugliese T, Soria A, Francès C, et al. Cutaneous drug-induced lupus erythematosus: clinical and immunological characteristics and update on new associated drugs. Ann Dermatol Venereol. 2021;148(4):211–20.
13. Szczęch J, Samotij D, Werth VP, Reich A. Trigger factors of cutaneous lupus erythematosus: a review of current literature. Lupus. 2017;26(8):791–807.
14. Lipsker D. The need to revisit the nosology of cutaneous lupus erythematosus: the current terminology and morphologic classification of cutaneous LE: difficult, incomplete and not always applicable. Lupus. 2010;19(9):1047–9.
15. Lin JH, Dutz JP, Sontheimer RD, Werth VP. Pathophysiology of cutaneous lupus erythematosus. Clin Rev Allergy Immunol. 2007;33(1–2):85–106.
16. Filotico R, Mastrandrea V. Cutaneous lupus erythematosus: clinico-pathologic correlation. G Ital Dermatol Venereol. 2018;153(2):216–29.
17. Wieczorek IT, Propert KJ, Okawa J, Werth VP. Systemic symptoms in the progression of cutaneous to systemic lupus erythematosus. JAMA Dermatol. 2014;150(3):291–6.
18. Grönhagen CM, Fored CM, Granath F, Nyberg F. Cutaneous lupus erythematosus and the association with systemic lupus erythematosus: a population-based cohort of 1088 patients in Sweden. Br J Dermatol. 2011;164(6):1335–41.
19. Mirali S, Mufti A, Lansang RP, Sachdeva M, Yeung J. Development of chronic cutaneous lupus erythematosus during biologic therapy: a systematic review. J Am Acad Dermatol. 2021;84(3):835–8.
20. Uva L, Miguel D, Pinheiro C, Freitas JP, Marques Gomes M, Filipe P. Cutaneous manifestations of

systemic lupus erythematosus. Autoimmune Dis. 2012:834291.
21. Kuhn A, Landmann A. The classification and diagnosis of cutaneous lupus erythematosus. J Autoimmun. 2014;48–49:14–9.
22. Sticherling M. [Cutaneous lupus erythematosus and skin manifestations in systemic lupus erythematosus]. Z Rheumatol. 2013;72(5):429–35.
23. Patel P, Werth V. Cutaneous lupus erythematosus: a review. Dermatol Clin. 2002;20(3):373–85.
24. Cooper EE, Pisano CE, Shapiro SC. Cutaneous manifestations of "lupus": systemic lupus erythematosus and beyond. Int J Rheumatol. 2021;2021:6610509.
25. Sunderkötter CH, Zelger B, Chen K-R, Requena L, Piette W, Carlson JA, et al. Nomenclature of cutaneous vasculitis: dermatologic addendum to the 2012 revised international chapel hill consensus conference nomenclature of vasculitides. Arthritis Rheumatol. 2018;70(2):171–84.
26. Udompanich S, Chanprapaph K, Suchonwanit P. Hair and scalp changes in cutaneous and systemic lupus erythematosus. Am J Clin Dermatol. 2018;19(5):679–94.
27. Zahn S, Rehkämper C, Kümmerer BM, Ferring-Schmidt S, Bieber T, Tüting T, et al. Evidence for a pathophysiological role of keratinocyte-derived type III interferon (IFNλ) in cutaneous lupus erythematosus. J Invest Dermatol. 2011;131(1):133–40.
28. Sarkar MK, Hile GA, Tsoi LC, Xing X, Liu J, Liang Y, et al. Photosensitivity and type I IFN responses in cutaneous lupus are driven by epidermal-derived interferon kappa. Ann Rheum Dis. 2018;77(11):1653–64.
29. Dey-Rao R, Sinha AA. Genome-wide transcriptional profiling data from skin of chronic cutaneous lupus erythematosus (CCLE) patients. Data Brief. 2015;4:47–9.
30. Scholtissek B, Zahn S, Maier J, Klaeschen S, Braegelmann C, Hoelzel M, et al. Immunostimulatory endogenous nucleic acids drive the lesional inflammation in cutaneous lupus erythematosus. J Invest Dermatol. 2017;137(7):1484–92.
31. Sinha AA, Dey-Rao R. Genomic investigation of lupus in the skin. J Investig Dermatol Symp Proc. 2017;18(2):S75–80.
32. Peschke K, Friebe F, Zimmermann N, Wahlicht T, Schumann T, Achleitner M, et al. Deregulated type I IFN response in TREX1-associated familial chilblain lupus. J Invest Dermatol. 2014;134(5):1456–9.
33. Hersh AO, Arkin LM, Prahalad S. Immunogenetics of cutaneous lupus erythematosus. Curr Opin Pediatr. 2016;28(4):470–5.
34. Curran CS, Gupta S, Sanz I, Sharon E. PD-1 immunobiology in systemic lupus erythematosus. J Autoimmun. 2019;97:1–9.
35. Fiorentino DF. The Yin and Yang of TNF-α inhibition. Arch Dermatol. 2007;143(2).
36. Shovman O, Tamar S, Amital H, Watad A, Shoenfeld Y. Diverse patterns of anti-TNF-α-induced lupus: case series and review of the literature. Clin Rheumatol. 2018;37(2):563–8.
37. Biermann MHC, Veissi S, Maueröder C, Chaurio R, Berens C, Herrmann M, et al. The role of dead cell clearance in the etiology and pathogenesis of systemic lupus erythematosus: dendritic cells as potential targets. Expert Rev Clin Immunol. 2014;10(9):1151–64.
38. Sandholdt LH, Laurinaviciene R, Bygum A. Proton pump inhibitor-induced subacute cutaneous lupus erythematosus. Br J Dermatol. 2014;170(2):342–51.
39. Vaglio A, Grayson PC, Fenaroli P, Gianfreda D, Boccaletti V, Ghiggeri GM, et al. Drug-induced lupus: traditional and new concepts. Autoimmun Rev. 2018;17(9):912–8.
40. Sharma A, Ahmad Farouk I, Lal SK. COVID-19: a review on the novel coronavirus disease evolution, transmission, detection, control and prevention. Viruses. 2021;13(2).
41. Msemburi W, Karlinsky A, Knutson V, Aleshin-Guendel S, Chatterji S, Wakefield J. The WHO estimates of excess mortality associated with the COVID-19 pandemic. Nature. 2023;613(7942):130–7.
42. Stokes EK, Zambrano LD, Anderson KN, Marder EP, Raz KM, El Burai Felix S, et al. Coronavirus disease 2019 case surveillance—United States, January 22-May 30, 2020. MMWR Morb Mortal Wkly Rep. 2020;69(24):759–65.
43. Bellan M, Apostolo D, Albè A, Crevola M, Errica N, Ratano G, et al. Determinants of long COVID among adults hospitalized for SARS-CoV-2 infection: a prospective cohort study. Front Immunol. 2022;13:1038227.
44. Matar S, Oulès B, Sohier P, Chosidow O, Beylot-Barry M, Dupin N, et al. Cutaneous manifestations in SARS-CoV-2 infection (COVID-19): a French experience and a systematic review of the literature. J Eur Acad Dermatol Venereol. 2020;34(11):e686–9.
45. Rajan MB, Kumar-M P, Bhardwaj A. The trend of cutaneous lesions during COVID-19 pandemic: lessons from a meta-analysis and systematic review. Int J Dermatol. 2020;59(11):1358–70.
46. Mande P, Zirak B, Ko W-C, Taravati K, Bride KL, Brodeur TY, et al. Fas ligand promotes an inducible TLR-dependent model of cutaneous lupus-like inflammation. J Clin Invest. 2018;128(7):2966–78.
47. Gao Z, Zhai X, Yan G, Tian Y, Huang X, Wu Q, et al. Bioinformatics analyses of gene expression profile to identify pathogenic mechanisms for COVID-19 infection and cutaneous lupus erythematosus. Front Immunol. 2023;14:1268912.
48. Petrea Cliveți CL, Ciortea D-A, Miulescu M, Candussi I-L, Chirila SI, Verga Răuță GI, et al. A new case of paediatric systemic lupus erythematosus with onset after SARS-CoV-2 and Epstein-Barr infection-a case report and literature review. Curr Issues Mol Biol. 2024;46(8):8642–57.
49. Nln I, Fernandez-Ruiz R, Muskardin TLW, Paredes JL, Blazer AD, Tuminello S, et al. Interferon pathway lupus risk alleles modulate risk of death from acute COVID-19. Transl Res. 2022;244:47–55.
50. Tsoi LC, Hile GA, Berthier CC, Sarkar MK, Reed TJ, Liu J, et al. Hypersensitive IFN responses in lupus

keratinocytes reveal key mechanistic determinants in cutaneous lupus. J Immunol. 2019;202(7):2121–30.
51. Xiang M, Chen Q, Feng Y, Wang Y, Wang J, Liang J, et al. Bioinformatic analysis of key biomarkers and immune filtration of skin biopsy in discoid lupus erythematosus. Lupus. 2021;30(5):807–17.
52. Yin X, Riva L, Pu Y, Martin-Sancho L, Kanamune J, Yamamoto Y, et al. MDA5 governs the innate immune response to SARS-CoV-2 in lung epithelial cells. Cell Rep. 2021;34(2):108628.
53. Zahn S, Barchet W, Rehkämper C, Hornung T, Bieber T, Tüting T, et al. Enhanced skin expression of melanoma differentiation-associated gene 5 (MDA5) in dermatomyositis and related autoimmune diseases. J Am Acad Dermatol. 2011;64(5):988–9.
54. Vishnubalaji R, Shaath H, Alajez NM. Protein Coding and Long Noncoding RNA (lncRNA) transcriptional landscape in SARS-CoV-2 infected bronchial epithelial cells highlight a role for interferon and inflammatory response. Genes. 2020;11(7).
55. Abuhammad A, AbuKhalaf SM, AbuKhalaf MM, Janem AM, Attawna SIY. Lupus panniculitis as the initial presentation of systemic lupus erythematosus triggered by COVID-19 infection: case report and literature review. Oxf Med Case Rep. 2023;2023(11):omad129.
56. Nunes AL, Simoes L, Figueiredo C, Carvalho R, Lima J, Santos RM. Toxic epidermal necrolysis-like lupus erythematous presentation following SARS-CoV-2 infection. J Med Cases. 2022;13(2):89–93.
57. Battesti G, El Khalifa J, Abdelhedi N, Ferre V, Bouscarat F, Picard-Dahan C, et al. New insights in COVID-19–associated chilblains: a comparative study with chilblain lupus erythematosus. J Am Acad Dermatol. 2020;83(4):1219–22.
58. Drenovska K, Shahid M, Mateeva V, Vassileva S. Case report: Rowell syndrome–like flare of cutaneous lupus erythematosus following COVID-19 infection. Front Med (Lausanne). 2022;9.
59. Barbagallo M, Straumann D, Binaghi E, Schmick A. A rare case of a wall-eyed bilateral internuclear ophthalmoplegia (WEBINO) syndrome in a patient with cutaneous lupus erythematosus after COVID-19 infection. J Neurol. 2023;270(3):1224–8.
60. Hadj Hassine I. Covid-19 vaccines and variants of concern: a review. Rev Med Virol. 2022;32(4):e2313.
61. https://covid19.who.int. [Internet]. [cited 2024 Sep 24]. Available from: https://covid19.who.int
62. Joseph AK, Chong BF. Subacute cutaneous lupus erythematosus flare triggered by COVID-19 vaccine. Dermatol Ther. 2021;34(6):e15114.
63. Liu V, Messenger NB. New-onset cutaneous lupus erythematosus after the COVID-19 vaccine. Dermatol Online J. 2021;27(11).
64. Zengarini C, Pileri A, Salamone FP, Piraccini BM, Vitale G, La Placa M. Subacute cutaneous lupus erythematosus induction after SARS-CoV-2 vaccine in a patient with primary biliary cholangitis. J Eur Acad Dermatol Venereol. 2022;36(3).
65. Niebel D, Ralser-Isselstein V, Jaschke K, Braegelmann C, Bieber T, Wenzel J. Exacerbation of subacute cutaneous lupus erythematosus following vaccination with BNT162b2 mRNA vaccine. Dermatol Ther. 2021;34(4):e15017.
66. Rechtien L, Erfurt-Berge C, Sticherling M. SCLE manifestation after mRNA COVID-19 vaccination. J Eur Acad Dermatol Venereol. 2022;36(4):e261–3.
67. Kreuter A, Burmann SN, Burkert B, Oellig F, Michalowitz AL. Transition of cutaneous into systemic lupus erythematosus following adenoviral vector-based SARS-CoV-2 vaccination. J Eur Acad Dermatol Venereol. 2021;35(11):e733–5.
68. Kreuter A, Licciardi-Fernandez MJ, Burmann SN, Burkert B, Oellig F, Michalowitz AL. Induction and exacerbation of subacute cutaneous lupus erythematosus following mRNA-based or adenoviral vector-based SARS-CoV-2 vaccination. Clin Exp Dermatol. 2022;47(1):161–3.
69. Rose C, Apgar R, Green M. Cutaneous lupus-erythematosus-like reaction arising after COVID-19 vaccination. J Cutan Pathol. 2022;49(11):943–6.
70. Bakr F, Denny J, Babakinejad P, Giles A, du Peloux Menagé H. Cutaneous lupus erythematosus flare with vitiligo-like depigmentation following the AstraZeneca COVID vaccine. JAAD Case Rep. 2022;30:51–5.
71. Nakahara Y, Yamane M, Sunada M, Aoyama Y. SARS-CoV-2 vaccine-triggered conversion from systemic lupus erythematosus (SLE) to bullous SLE and dipeptidyl peptidase 4 inhibitors-associated bullous pemphigoid. J Dermatol. 2023;50(2):162–5.
72. Rimmer S, Ly L, Boh E. Subacute cutaneous lupus erythematosus after mRNA-based SARS-CoV-2 vaccination. JAAD Case Rep. 2023;33:70–2.
73. Famularo G, Patti AL, Macciomei MC. COVID-19 vaccine-induced cutaneous lupus erythematosus. Dermatol Online J. 2023;29(5).
74. Souza EN, Diniz LM, Moura LA, Oliosi AC. Exacerbation of chronic cutaneous lupus erythematosus triggered by vaccine against COVID-19. Actas Dermosifiliogr. 2024;115(4):430–2.
75. Pour Mohammad A, Noroozi E, Mesgarha MG, Shayanfar N, Goodarzi A. Interesting mucocutaneous manifestations in COVID-19 infection or vaccination confirmed by histopathology: a case series. Case Rep Dermatol. 2024;16(1):21–34.
76. Vezzoli P, Di Mercurio M, Carugno A, Gambini DM, Robustelli Test E, Imberti G, et al. Cutaneous lupus erythematosus patients in a high-epidemic COVID-19 area, Bergamo, Italy. Dermatol Ther. 2020;33(4):e13776.

5 The Effect of COVID-19 and Its Vaccination on Lichen Planus Exacerbation

Maleehah Faatimah, N. L. Swathi, Rajeswari Madishetty, Md. Ayesha Sultana, Chittepu Charankumar Reddy, Sangeetha komma, and Esraa M. AlEdani

5.1 Introduction: Overview of Lichen Planus and COVID-19

5.1.1 Background of Lichen Planus (LP)

Lichen Planus (LP) is a chronic inflammatory condition affecting about 1% of the global population, primarily affecting the skin and mucous membranes. It is present in various forms, including cutaneous and oral, and significantly affects the patients' quality of life. The pathogenesis of LP is multifaceted, with common triggers including hepatitis C virus (HCV) infection, mechanical trauma, psychological stress, and microbiota abnormalities. Immunopathogenesis is primarily influenced by cell-mediated cytotoxicity, including cytotoxic T lymphocytes and Th1 and IL-23/Th-17 pathways. Immune cells and inflammatory pathways also play a role [1].

Immune-mediated processes account for most of the pathophysiology of LP, with cell-mediated cytotoxicity against basal keratinocytes coordinated by cytotoxic T lymphocytes. The immune response in LP lesions is further enhanced by the Th1 and IL-23/Th-17 axes, which contribute to the inflammatory environment. Environmental factors such as HCV infection can be linked to LP, with patients with LP having varying levels of HCV prevalence. Psychological stress and mechanical trauma are common precipitants that may act by rupturing mucosal barriers and triggering the immune system [1].

The components of metabolic syndrome are known to occur more frequently in LP patients, suggesting a potential interaction between chronic inflammation and systemic metabolic dysregulation [2]. Aryanian et al. [2] reported increased concentrations of leptin and C-reactive protein (CRP) in patients with LP relative to healthy controls; however, the study's cross-sectional methodology constrains causal interpretations.

The caliber of the evidence among the examined papers was inconsistent. The prevalence of

M. Faatimah (✉)
Department of Pharmaceutical Sciences, MRM College of Pharmacy, Jawaharlal Nehru Technological University, Hyderabad, Telangana, India

N. L. Swathi · C. C. Reddy
Department of Pharmacy Practice, Jawaharlal Nehru Technology University, Anantapur, Andhra Pradesh, India

R. Madishetty
Malla Reddy Institute of Pharmaceutical Sciences, Hyderabad, Telangana, India

M. Ayesha Sultana · S. komma
Nirmala College of Pharmacy, Autonomous, Guntur District, Andhra Pradesh, India

E. M. AlEdani
University of Basrah-Medical Faculty, Basrah, Iraq

E. M. AlEdani, H. Maibach (eds.), *COVID-19 Vaccination and Dermatological Diseases*, Updates in Clinical Dermatology, https://doi.org/10.1007/978-3-031-87791-9_5

narrative reviews offers extensive summaries but frequently lacks the methodological rigor found in systematic reviews or meta-analyses. The original research conducted by Aryanian et al. [2] provides empirical evidence; nevertheless, it is constrained by its cross-sectional design and the small sample size of 40 LP patients. The case series by Erthal et al. [3] offers clinical insights, but is fundamentally constrained by its retrospective design and the possibility of selection bias. The conference report by Chang et al. [4] provides insights on associated inflammatory disorders but presents limited empirical data specifically about LP.

Statistical investigations indicate that LP primarily affects middle-aged females, exhibiting a chronic trajectory marked by recurring flare-ups [1, 3, 5, 6]. The correlation between LP and HCV is especially significant in areas with elevated HCV prevalence, highlighting the necessity for regular screening of LP patients exhibiting risk indicators [7, 8]. Moreover, the risk of malignant development in LP, especially in mucosal variants, underscores the importance of diligent surveillance and prompt intervention [3, 6].

5.1.2 Introduction to COVID-19

The COVID-19 pandemic, induced by the SARS-CoV-2 virus, has significantly affected world health since its onset in late 2019. This respiratory ailment has a spectrum of severity, ranging from asymptomatic to severe pneumonia and mortality. Comprehending COVID-19 requires an analysis of its transmission, clinical presentations, diagnostic techniques, and treatment approaches.

The transmission of SARS-CoV-2 predominantly occurs via respiratory droplets, rendering interventions such as mask usage, hand cleanliness, and physical distancing, which are essential for mitigating its dissemination. Vaccination is a crucial strategy for alleviating this pandemic. Multiple vaccines, such as mRNA (e.g., Pfizer-BioNTech, Moderna), viral vectors (e.g., AstraZeneca, Janssen), and inactivated vaccines (e.g., Sinovac) have been created and distributed worldwide. These vaccinations have exhibited differing levels of effectiveness against several variants of concern (VOCs) including Delta and Omicron [9, 10].

Research demonstrates that whereas vaccinations are exceptionally successful in preventing severe illness and hospitalization, their efficacy against infection and symptomatic disease may diminish with time, particularly with the development of novel variations [9, 11, 12]. Booster dosages have demonstrated the ability to augment protection, especially against variants of concern such as Delta and Omicron. Furthermore, immunization has been linked to a diminished likelihood of developing protracted COVID, a syndrome characterized by enduring symptoms following infection [13, 14].

Diagnostic methodologies for COVID-19 have progressed, with RT-PCR being recognized as the gold standard for detection owing to its high specificity, despite drawbacks such as false negatives and the requirement for specialized laboratory environments [15, 16]. Rapid antigen tests provide expedited findings, but are typically less sensitive. Imaging modalities, especially chest CT scans, contribute to evaluating disease severity but are not exclusively dependable for diagnosis [15].

The management of COVID-19 mainly entails supportive treatment, encompassing oxygen therapy and mechanical breathing for critical cases. Antiviral agents such as remdesivir and immunomodulatory therapies, including corticosteroids, have been used to enhance patient outcomes [17, 18]. Preventive interventions in conjunction with immunization are crucial for mitigating viral transmission [19].

The advent of SARS-CoV-2 mutations highlights the need for ongoing surveillance and modification of public health initiatives. Vaccines have demonstrated considerable effectiveness against variants of concern (VOCs) however, certain variants may show diminished efficiency, underscoring the necessity for booster doses and the advancement of next-generation vaccines [9, 10]. Moreover, particular demographics, such as pregnant women and children, have been rigorously examined to ascertain vaccine safety and efficacy in various populations [12, 20].

Studying the impact of COVID-19 and its vaccines on Lichen Planus (LP) exacerbation is crucial for patient care and public health, particularly in the context of autoimmune diseases. The immune dysregulation and inflammation of the virus could provide insights into how viral infections interact with autoimmune diseases, helping clinicians manage flare-ups in patients with LP. This study also raises concerns about the safety of vaccination in individuals with autoimmune conditions. Understanding the interplay among COVID-19, vaccines, and LP is vital for creating informed health policies and tailoring vaccination strategies for at-risk populations. Future research could enhance the preventive and therapeutic strategies for managing LP in the COVID-19 era.

5.2 Pathophysiology of Lichen Planus and Immune Response to COVID-19

1. **Immunopathogenesis of Lichen Planus**

Lichen Planus is a persistent disorder that impacts the skin and mucous membranes, including the oral cavity. This induces inflammation and may result in painful ulcers and lesions. The immune system, specifically the T cells, is pivotal in the pathogenesis of Lichen Planus. The pathogenesis of Lichen Planus is primarily influenced by T cell-mediated immunological responses, especially those involving CD8 + cytotoxic T lymphocytes and mucosal-associated invariant T (MAIT) cells. These T cells induce immunological dysregulation by secreting pro-inflammatory cytokines, including TNF-α and IFN-γ, which results in keratinocyte death and persistent inflammatory lesions. A weakness in regulatory mechanisms, such as TGF-β1-mediated immunosuppression, exacerbates the chronicity of the disease, underscoring a complex interaction between immunological activation and regulatory failure in the immunopathogenesis of Lichen Planus.

T cells are crucial for protecting the body from infections and various disorders. In Lichen Planus, these cells erroneously target and assault the body's own tissues. This aberrant immune response results in the obliteration of cells in impacted regions, eliciting hallmark signs of the disease (Fig. 5.1).

Studies have indicated that both specific and non-specific immunological mechanisms play a role in Lichen Planus pathogenesis. Particular mechanisms entail T-cell identification and attachment to specific antigens (foreign substances) present on the surface of the skin or mucosal cells. Upon activation, these T-cells secrete chemicals that eliminate targeted cells [21]. Conversely, non-specific pathways involve the secretion of enzymes and inflammatory mediators that further injure tissues and intensify inflammation [22]. The immunopathogenesis of lichen anus (LP) is intricately governed by T cell subsets and is marked by immunological dysregulation, as detailed in the reviewed literature. Sugerman et al. (2002) elucidate the crucial function of $CD8^{+}$ cytotoxic T lymphocytes in attacking basal keratinocytes, hence promoting antigen-specific keratinocyte death [22]. The cytotoxic action is exacerbated by non-specific inflammatory processes, such as mast cell degranulation and the activation of matrix metalloproteinases (MMPs), which together compromise the basement membrane and sustain T cell infiltration. The aggregation of T cells in the superficial lamina propria and their translocation into intra-epithelial areas indicates a vigorous adaptive immune response that supports lesion formation [22].

Moreover, specific specialized T-cells, including mucosal-associated invariant T (MAIT) cells, may contribute to the immunological dysregulation observed in Lichen Planus. These cells are generally engaged in the body's response to microbial infections but may also play a role in aberrant immunological activity that results in tissue damage in this illness [21]. DeAngelis et al. (2019) elucidate the role of mucosal-associated invariant T (MAIT) cells in oral lichen planus, thereby broadening the immunological framework beyond traditional T-cell subsets [21]. MAIT cells, recognized for their function in antimicrobial defense, may influence the inflammatory environment of LP through their

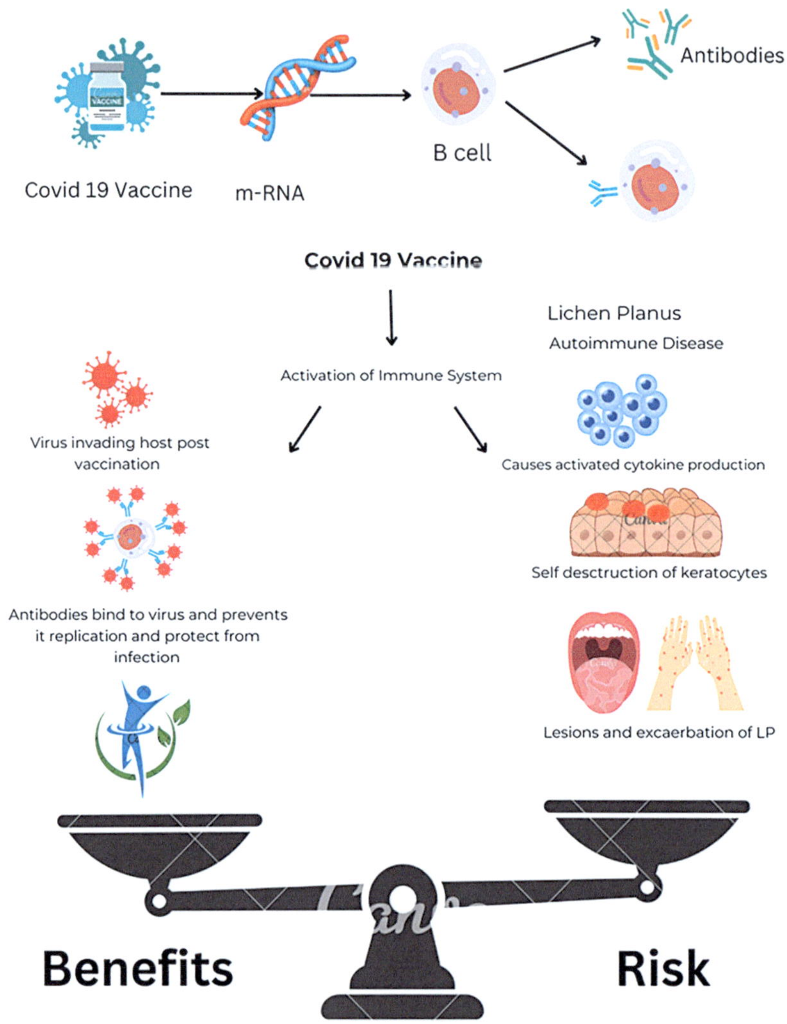

Fig. 5.1 Effect of covid 19 vaccination on lichen planus: risks and benefits

rapid cytokine production, including IFN-γ and TNF-α, thereby enhancing immune responses and facilitating epithelial damage. The connection between MAIT cells and oral microbiota indicates a potential environmental trigger that, together with host susceptibility characteristics, begins and perpetuates the chronic inflammatory condition seen in LP [21].

Environmental variables, genetic predisposition, and potential disturbances in the oral microbiota are thought to elicit aberrant T cell responses in individuals predisposed to Lichen Planus. The persistent nature of the disease may originate from continuous immune system activation and breakdown of regulatory mechanisms that typically regulate T cell activity.

The immunopathogenesis of Lichen Planus involves a complicated interaction between T cell-mediated immune responses and immune system abnormalities. Understanding these pathways is essential for formulating tailored medicines to manage and treat this illness successfully.

Both investigations highlighted the disparity between pro-inflammatory cytokines and regulatory factors in the pathophysiology of LP. Sugerman et al. emphasized a shortcoming of TGF-β1-mediated immunosuppression, which is essential for sustaining immunological homeostasis and averting excessive inflammatory reactions [2]. This deficit permits unregulated T cell activity and prolonged cytokine production, resulting in ongoing tissue injury and lesion persistence [22].

The disruption of immune privilege in the oral mucosa, possibly similar to other immuno-privileged regions, including the eye and testis, promotes abnormal immune surveillance and autoimmunity [22].

The quality of evidence in these reviews is mainly derived from observational studies and experimental models, and Sugerman et al. incorporated results from immunohistochemical analysis and clinical correlations in a cohort of patients diagnosed with oral LP [22]. While both articles offer thorough examinations of the immunological pathways in LP, their dependence on preclinical and correlational data inevitably constrains the robustness of the causal findings. DeAngelis et al. (2019) integrated new findings on MAIT cell biology; however, the introduction of MAIT cells requires additional empirical validation through focused research to confirm their function in the LP [21].

The immunopathogenesis of Lichen Planus is mostly based on T cell-mediated processes and notable immunological dysregulation. CD8 + cytotoxic T cells are pivotal for targeting and causing apoptosis in basal keratinocytes, thereby directly facilitating lesion formation. Recent findings regarding MAIT cells have enhanced our understanding of the T-cell milieu in LP, indicating that these cells may potentiate inflammatory responses via cytokine production following engagement with the oral microbiota. Furthermore, the persistence of LP can be ascribed to a disparity between pro-inflammatory cytokines and regulatory elements such as TGF-β1, resulting in prolonged immune activation and tissue injury. The disruption of immune privilege in the oral mucosa intensifies this dysregulation, facilitating the ongoing and repeated formation of lesions. These results highlight the intricacy of T-cell interactions and the need for tailored therapy techniques that focus on both the activation of pathogenic T cells and the restoration of immune regulatory mechanisms in the management of Lichen Planus.

2. **Immune Response to SARS-CoV-2**

COVID-19 induces a multifaceted immune response that can lead to severe inflammatory events such as a cytokine storm, potentially aggravating autoimmune disorders such as lichen planus (LP). Understanding the mechanisms underlying this relationship is crucial for understanding how COVID-19, via both infection and vaccination, may affect LP flareups.

5.2.1 Cytokine Storm in COVID-19

SARS-CoV-2, which is responsible for COVID-19, may trigger an excessive immune response in certain patients, resulting in a phenomenon termed cytokine storm. A cytokine storm is a hyperinflammatory condition marked by the overproduction of pro-inflammatory cytokines such as interleukin-6 (IL-6), tumor necrosis factor-alpha (TNF-α), and interferon-gamma (IFN-γ). These cytokines are essential in modulating immune responses; nevertheless, excessive production can result in extensive tissue damage, multi-organ failure, and serious consequences, such as acute respiratory distress syndrome (ARDS), thrombosis, and vasculitis [23].The onset of a cytokine storm in COVID-19 patients is frequently associated with the virus's engagement with angiotensin-converting enzyme 2 (ACE2) receptors, which are present in multiple cell types, including alveolar epithelial cells in the lungs, endothelial cells, and cardiac and renal cells. Following viral entry, the body initiates a robust immunological response that engages both the innate and adaptive immune systems. This response may occasionally become dysregulated, resulting in a delayed or ineffective type I interferon response that fails to eliminate the virus, thereby permitting excessive inflammation [24].

5.2.2 Immunopathogenesis of Lichen Planus

Lichen planus is an autoimmune condition driven by T cells that attack basal keratinocytes in the skin and mucous membranes, resulting in distinctive LP lesions. Immunological dysregulation observed in LP, especially the imbalance between Th1 and Th2, includes pro-inflammatory cytokines, including IFN-γ, TNF-α, and IL-6, which are also associated with cytokine storms in COVID-19. The convergence of immunological pathways indicates that the inflammatory milieu induced by COVID-19 infection, or by the immune response elicited by vaccination, may aggravate LP in susceptible patients.

Research indicates an increase in the exacerbations of oral lichen planus (OLP) and new cases of lichen planus subsequent to COVID-19 infection or immunization, particularly with mRNA vaccines. The increased inflammatory conditions during or following infection may enhance the production of the same cytokines and immune cells that contribute to LP pathogenesis, potentially resulting in exacerbations in patients with pre-existing LP or initiating LP in those without prior disease. This mechanism is believed to encompass T-cell dysregulation and cross-reactivity between viral antigens and self-antigens, resulting in the activation of autoreactive T-cells [23].

5.2.3 Autoimmune Exacerbations in Lichen Planus Post-COVID-19

Extended immunological activation and systemic inflammation caused by cytokine storms during COVID-19 have been associated with autoimmune exacerbations in diseases, such as LP. Cytokine storms can directly affect the activity of autoimmune diseases through multiple mechanisms.

T-cell Exhaustion and Dysfunction: COVID-19 has demonstrated a reduction in both CD4+ and CD8+ T-cell populations, while elevating the levels of IL-6, TNF-α, and IL-10, thereby biasing the immune system towards an excessive yet ineffective response. The decrease in T-cell numbers is linked to illness severity and coincides with immunological exhaustion, as noted in [25]. Dysregulation of T-cells may trigger the re-emergence of autoimmune illnesses, such as LP, by permitting pro-inflammatory signals to remain unregulated.

Interleukin-6 (IL-6) is a key cytokine implicated in inflammation associated with COVID-19. Increased IL-6 levels have been recognized as an indicator of severe illness and unfavorable outcomes in COVID-19 patients, according to [24, 25]. IL-6 is also involved in the pathophysiology of autoimmune disorders including LP. This cytokine facilitates the differentiation of Th17 cells, which have been implicated in chronic inflammation and autoimmunity. The increase in IL-6 during a cytokine storm may exacerbate LP symptoms.

Molecular mimicry is a process in which the immune system erroneously targets self-tissues following stimulation by viral antigens that closely resemble the host antigens. This behavior has been associated with the aggravation of autoimmune illnesses subsequent to viral infections, and may explain why certain LP patients have flare-ups after catching COVID-19 [23].

5.2.4 Effects of COVID-19 Vaccination on Lichen Planus

COVID-19 vaccinations, particularly mRNA vaccines such as Pfizer-BioNTech and Moderna, have been linked to autoimmune flareups in certain instances, including exacerbations of lichen planus. Vaccines are intended to elicit a regulated immune response to generate antibodies against the virus; however, in rare instances, this stimulation may trigger autoimmune reactions in susceptible individuals [25, 26].

The mechanism by which immunization induces an LP flare is believed to be associated with activation of the immune system. Adjuvants in vaccinations, which are incorporated to augment the immunological response, may occasionally result in excessive immune activation in specific individuals. This over-activation may induce the release of cytokines implicated in the LP pathophysiology, resulting in exacerbation. Nonetheless, the advantages of immunization, especially in mitigating severe COVID-19, are far above the dangers of aggravating autoimmune disorders in the majority of cases [23].

5.3 Clinical Evidence of Lichen Planus Exacerbation Post-COVID-19 Infection

1. **Case Reports and Studies**

Exacerbations of lichen planus (LP) subsequent to COVID-19 have been documented in a number of case studies and case series published in medical journals. SARS-CoV-2 may cause immunological alterations that could result in LP flareups. LP is an inflammatory disease that primarily affects the skin and mucous membrane. The cases and series of recorded LP exacerbations that occurred after COVID-19 are included here along with links to pertinent research and review papers.

- **Case 1: Post-COVID-19 Infection Lichen Planus Flare (Egypt, 2021).**

Case Report: Two weeks after recovering from a mild COVID-19 infection, a 45-year-old male patient with oral lichen planus (OLP) experienced a major flare-up of his illness. The patient experienced erythema, ulceration, and painful oral lesions.

Treatment: Topical corticosteroids and immunomodulatory drugs were used to treat the exacerbation, which resulted in progressive improvement in symptoms.

Theory: Immunological dysregulation caused by SARS-CoV-2 might have triggered a T-cell-mediated reaction, which would have worsened LP [27].

- **Case 2: COVID-19 and Lichen Planus Exacerbation**

  Case Series:

- In a study from Turkey, three patients (aged 38–56 years) with a known history of cutaneous LP reported worsening of their skin lesions 3–4 weeks post-COVID-19 infection. The flare-ups presented as hypertrophic lesions, increased pruritus, and new sites of involvement including the oral mucosa.
- **Treatment**: Systemic corticosteroids and retinoids are required for symptom management.
- **Significance**: This case series suggests that viral infections, particularly COVID-19, might exacerbate pre-existing autoimmune conditions such as LP [3].

- **Case 3: Oral and Cutaneous Lichen Planus Exacerbation Post-COVID-19.**

  Case Report:

- After contracting COVID-19, a 58-year-old woman with a 10-year history of both oral and cutaneous LP presented with flare-up of both manifestations. She developed violaceous papules on her arms and legs, white reticular lesions on the buccal mucosa, and an increase in the oral burning sensation. The patient was treated with topical corticosteroids and tacrolimus for oral lesions, and systemic prednisone was initiated for cutaneous symptoms. This case illustrates how COVID-19 can alter the immune system and cause the disease to reactivate [28].

- **Case 4: COVID-19-Induced Exacerbation of Lichen Planopilaris.**

  Case Study:

- A 42-year-old female with a prior diagnosis of lichen planopilaris (LPP), a variant of LP affecting the scalp, experienced significant exacerbation of hair loss and scalp inflammation following a mild COVID-19 infection.
- **Findings**: Dermoscopy revealed perifollicular scaling and erythema, consistent with active LPP. The patient had stable LPP 3 years prior to COVID-19.
- **Hypothesis**: The study suggests that Viral-induced cytokine storms may worsen conditions such as LPP through immune dysregulation [29].

5.4 Impact of COVID-19 Vaccination on Lichen Planus: Safety and Exacerbation Risk

1. **Overview of COVID-19 Vaccines**

COVID-19 vaccines are instrumental in controlling the global pandemic by providing immunity against SARS-CoV-2. Various types of vaccines use different technologies to stimulate the immune system. mRNA vaccines contain a small piece of messenger RNA that instructs cells to produce a harmless spike protein similar to that found on the surface of the virus. These vaccines generate a strong immune response, including neutralizing antibodies and cellular immunity, which protects against infection and reduces disease severity [30].

Viral vector vaccines use a harmless virus modified to carry genetic material coding for the SARS-CoV-2 spike protein. Once the viral vector enters human cells, the cells begin to produce a spike protein, which triggers an immune response. These vaccines stimulate both humoral (antibody) and cellular (T cell) immune responses, thereby providing robust immunity against COVID-19. They are effective in preventing severe disease, hospitalization, and death, although they may have slightly lower efficacy than mRNA vaccines in preventing mild or moderate infections [31].

Protein subunit vaccines contain harmless pieces of SARS-CoV-2 virus, usually the spike protein, but not the entire virus. When the immune system encounters these proteins, it mounts a response by generating antibodies without the need for live virus or genetic material. These vaccines generate strong antibody responses and can be combined with adjuvants to improve their efficacies [30, 31].

Inactivated or attenuated virus vaccines use viruses that have been killed or weakened, so that they can no longer cause disease. They trigger a broad immune response, exposing the immune system to the entire virus and not just the spike protein. They are effective at preventing severe disease, although they may produce a weaker immune response than mRNA or viral vector vaccines, especially against new variants [32].

While all vaccines play a critical role in controlling the pandemic, the development of new variants has led to ongoing research on the long-term efficacy of vaccines and the potential need for booster doses to maintain immunity.

2. **Immune Mechanisms of Vaccine-Induced Exacerbation**

The immune mechanisms underlying vaccine-induced exacerbation of lichen planus (LP) involve a complex interplay of immune stimulation, vaccine adjuvants, and potential cross-reactivity. These mechanisms may lead to the reactivation or worsening of autoimmune conditions, such as LP, following vaccination, particularly COVID-19 vaccines.

1. **Immune Stimulation and Cytokine Release:** COVID-19 vaccines, especially mRNA and viral vector platforms, are designed to generate a strong immune response to the spike protein of SARS-CoV-2. This immune response involves both humoral (antibodies) and cellular (T-cell) mechanisms. LP is predominantly a T-cell mediated disease, and vaccines, particularly mRNA vaccines, elicit robust T-cell responses, including the production of pro-inflammatory cytokines, such as interferon-gamma (IFN-γ) and tumor necrosis factor-alpha (TNF-α) [31].
2. **Cytokine Storm and Immune Dysregulation:** In cases, COVID-19 vaccination can trigger a temporary "cytokine storm," where a surge in immune molecules such as IL-6, TNF-α, and IFN-γ contributes to systemic inflammation. This heightened immune state may exacerbate autoimmune conditions, including LP, by creating an environment in which autoreactive T-cells are activated or reactivated, amplifying the autoimmune response against skin or mucosal tissues [33].
3. **Adjuvants:** Many vaccines use adjuvants to enhance the immune response; however, these adjuvants can also influence autoimmune pathways. Molecular mimicry and cross-

reactivity can cause the immune system to mistakenly target self-antigens, thereby resulting in autoimmunity [34].

4. **Pre-existing Immune Dysregulation:** Individuals with autoimmune conditions, such as LP, may already have underlying immune dysregulation, such as an imbalance in regulatory T-cells (Tregs) and effector T-cells. Vaccination could further tilt the immune balance toward an inflammatory response, potentially overcoming the body's normal regulatory mechanisms and triggering disease exacerbation [34].
5. **Bystander activation** occurs when immune cells, particularly T cells, are activated by inflammatory signals, even in the absence of a specific antigen. Inflammation as a trigger: The immune system creates an environment rich in pro-inflammatory cytokines, which could inadvertently activate autoreactive T-cells present in LP, leading to worsening of the disease without direct involvement of the spike protein or adjuvants [35].

5.5 Management Strategies for Lichen Planus in the COVID-19 Era

Lichen planus (LP) is a chronic inflammatory autoimmune disorder that affects the skin, mucous membranes, hair follicles, and nail. It is mediated by T cells that target and destroy basal keratinocytes in the skin or mucosa, leading to characteristic lesions. The COVID-19 pandemic has posed unique challenges for individuals with LP as both infection and vaccination have been associated with disease exacerbations. With the global rollout of vaccines and continued infection rates, managing LP in the context of COVID-19 has become increasingly important.

Lichen planus is predominantly driven by a T cell-mediated immune response, which is exacerbated by the inflammatory environment created during viral infections, particularly COVID-19. The immune response to the virus involves the production of cytokines, such as interferon-gamma (IFN-γ) and tumor necrosis factor-alpha (TNF-α), which can further fuel autoimmune reactions, leading to LP exacerbations. Vaccines, especially mRNA and viral vector types, also trigger immune activation to build protection against the virus; however, this can occasionally provoke flares in individuals with autoimmune disorders [36].

Medical therapies for LP exacerbations include corticosteroids, calcineurin inhibitors, systemic immunosuppressants, biological therapies, and phototherapy. Corticosteroids are the cornerstone of treatment for LP exacerbations, whereas calcineurin inhibitors suppress the immune response locally and reduce inflammation without side effects. Systemic immunosuppressants, such as cyclosporine, methotrexate, and azathioprine, have been successfully used to control LP by dampening the overall immune response [37].

Biological therapies, particularly TNF inhibitors, have been explored in refractory cases of LP, targeting specific pathways in the immune system. However, their use in the context of COVID-19 and vaccination requires careful consideration because of the risk of infection [31].

Oral lichen planus (OLP) is a chronic form of LP that can be challenging to manage, particularly following COVID-19 or vaccination-related exacerbations. Treatment includes topical corticosteroids and immunosuppressants; systemic therapies may be required for erosive OLP. Case reports and observational studies have documented successful management of LP exacerbations following COVID-19 infection or vaccination. Most patients respond well to conventional treatments, whereas a minority may require systemic immunosuppressants.

Vaccination is essential for preventing severe disease, hospitalization, and death from COVID-19, but there are concerns about potential vaccine-induced flares. Balancing vaccination and autoimmune risk is crucial in patients with LP. COVID-19 vaccination is strongly recommended for patients with LP, as the risk of severe complications far outweighs the potential for a mild or moderate LP flare. Pre-vaccination counseling is important, and patients should be educated on recognizing early signs of LP flares, such as increased pruritus, new lesions, or worsening oral discomfort. Regular post-vaccination follow-up appointments can help catch and treat exacerbations early, preventing them from becoming more severe.

Strategies for reducing flare risk include premedication with low-dose corticosteroids or immunosuppressants prior to vaccination, dampening the immune response, and preventing flares. The timing of vaccination should be carefully considered, ideally when the disease is in remission or is well-controlled [36].

Future Directions and Research Needs
Notwithstanding these insights, substantial gaps persist in our understanding of the link between COVID-19, immunization, and LP. Further investigation is required to elucidate the immunological systems at play and to devise strategies for reducing flare risk in patients with autoimmune diseases.

Research Gap
A significant gap exists in the absence of extensive studies examining the incidence of LP flares after vaccination. Existing data are primarily derived from case reports and limited observational research, constraining our capacity to generalize the findings. Comprehending the actual prevalence of vaccine-induced LP exacerbations and identifying at-risk populations are essential steps.

Research Priorities
Longitudinal investigations: Creating registries of patients with LP to monitor disease activity prior to and during vaccination or COVID-19
Immunological mechanisms: Examine the precise immunological processes implicated in vaccine-induced exacerbations, including T-cell activation and cytokine patterns.
Optimization of treatment: Assessing the effectiveness of novel medicines, including JAK inhibitors, in controlling LP exacerbations following immunization.

Personalized treatment may help to reduce the risk of LP. By identifying biomarkers that forecast flare risk, immunization regimens and therapies can be customized for individual patients, thereby reducing their risk of exacerbation and enhancing protection against COVID-19 [36].

5.6 Conclusion

The link between COVID-19 and lichen planus (LP) highlights the importance of vaccination in preventing severe illness and hospitalization. However, the risk of exacerbating LP outweighs the benefits. The personalized management of LP exacerbations requires corticosteroids, immunosuppressants, and biological therapies. Prioritizing pre-vaccination counseling and optimizing vaccination timing are crucial. Further research is needed to understand the immunological mechanisms linking COVID-19, vaccination, and LP and to develop targeted therapies.

References

1. Vičić M, Hlača N, Kaštelan M, Brajac I, Sotošek V, Prpić ML. Comprehensive Insight into Lichen Planus Immunopathogenesis. Int J Mol Sci. 2023;24(3):3038.
2. Aryanian Z, Shirzadian A, Hatami P, Dadras H. High incidence of metabolic syndrome components in Lichen Planus patients: a prospective cross-sectional study. Int J Clin Pract. 2022;2022:7184678.
3. Erthal A, Lourenço SV, Nico MMS. Oral lichen planus: case series and experience in a tertiary dermatology service in Brazil. An Bras Dermatol. 2023;98(4):493–7.
4. Chang WC, Abe R, Anderson P, Anderson W, Ardern-Jones MR, Beachkofsky TM, et al. SJS/TEN 2019: from science to translation. J Dermatol Sci. 2020;98(1):2–12.
5. Gorouhi F, Davari P, Fazel N. Cutaneous and mucosal lichen planus: a comprehensive review of clinical subtypes, risk factors, diagnosis, and prognosis. ScientificWorldJournal. 2014;2014:742826.
6. Ismail SB, Kumar SKS, Zain RB. Oral lichen planus and lichenoid reactions: etiopathogenesis, diagnosis, management and malignant transformation. J Oral Sci. 2007;49(2):89–106.
7. Dedania B, Wu GY. Dermatologic extrahepatic manifestations of hepatitis C. J Clin Transl Hepatol. 2015;3(2):127–33.
8. Georgescu SR, Tampa M, Mitran MI, Mitran CI, Sarbu MI, Nicolae I, et al. Potential pathogenic mech-

anisms involved in the association between lichen planus and hepatitis C virus infection. Exp Ther Med. 2019;17(2):1045–51.
9. Rahmati M, Yon DK, Lee SW, Butler L, Koyanagi A, Jacob L, et al. Effects of COVID-19 vaccination during pregnancy on SARS-CoV-2 infection and maternal and neonatal outcomes: a systematic review and meta-analysis. Rev Med Virol. 2023;33(3):e2434.
10. Zeng B, Gao L, Zhou Q, Yu K, Sun F. Effectiveness of COVID-19 vaccines against SARS-CoV-2 variants of concern: a systematic review and meta-analysis. BMC Med. 2022;20(1):200.
11. Dr F, Mm H, Lj AR, et al. Duration of effectiveness of vaccines against SARS-CoV-2 infection and COVID-19 disease: results of a systematic review and meta-regression. Lancet (London, England) [Internet]. 2022 [cited 2024 Oct 12];399(10328). Available from: https://pubmed.ncbi.nlm.nih.gov/35202601/
12. Ceban F, Ling S, Lui LMW, Lee Y, Gill H, Teopiz KM, et al. Fatigue and cognitive impairment in post-COVID-19 syndrome: a systematic review and meta-analysis. Brain Behav Immun. 2022;101:93–135.
13. Watanabe A, Iwagami M, Yasuhara J, Takagi H, Kuno T. Protective effect of COVID-19 vaccination against long COVID syndrome: a systematic review and meta-analysis. Vaccine. 2023;41(11):1783–90.
14. Talic S, Shah S, Wild H, Gasevic D, Maharaj A, Ademi Z, et al. Effectiveness of public health measures in reducing the incidence of covid-19, SARS-CoV-2 transmission, and covid-19 mortality: systematic review and meta-analysis. BMJ. 2021;375:e068302.
15. Yüce M, Filiztekin E, Özkaya KG. COVID-19 diagnosis -a review of current methods. Biosens Bioelectron. 2021;172:112752.
16. Cui X, Zhao Z, Zhang T, Guo W, Guo W, Zheng J, et al. A systematic review and meta-analysis of children with coronavirus disease 2019 (COVID-19). J Med Virol. 2021;93(2):1057–69.
17. Umakanthan S, Sahu P, Ranade AV, Bukelo MM, Rao JS, Abrahao-Machado LF, et al. Origin, transmission, diagnosis and management of coronavirus disease 2019 (COVID-19). Postgrad Med J. 2020;96(1142):753–8.
18. Majumder J, Minko T. Recent developments on therapeutic and diagnostic approaches for COVID-19. AAPS J. 2021;23(1):14.
19. Feikin DR, Higdon MM, Abu-Raddad LJ, Andrews N, Araos R, Goldberg Y, et al. Duration of effectiveness of vaccines against SARS-CoV-2 infection and COVID-19 disease: results of a systematic review and meta-regression. Lancet. 2022;399(10328):924–44.
20. Fernandes Q, Inchakalody VP, Merhi M, Mestiri S, Taib N, Moustafa Abo El-Ella D, et al. Emerging COVID-19 variants and their impact on SARS-CoV-2 diagnosis, therapeutics and vaccines. Ann Med. 2022;54(1):524–40.
21. DeAngelis LM, Cirillo N, McCullough MJ. The immunopathogenesis of oral lichen planus-Is there a role for mucosal associated invariant T cells? J Oral Pathol Med. 2019;48(7):552–9.
22. Sugerman PB, Savage NW, Walsh LJ, Zhao ZZ, Zhou XJ, Khan A, et al. The pathogenesis of oral lichen planus. Crit Rev Oral Biol Med. 2002;13(4):350–65.
23. Zou H, Daveluy S. Lichen planus after COVID-19 infection and vaccination. Arch Dermatol Res. 2023;315(2):139–46.
24. Bhaskar S, Sinha A, Banach M, Mittoo S, Weissert R, Kass JS, et al. Cytokine storm in COVID-19—immunopathological mechanisms, clinical considerations, and therapeutic approaches: the REPROGRAM consortium position paper. Front Immunol [Internet]. 2020 [cited 2024 Oct 12];11. Available from: https://www.frontiersin.org/journals/immunology/articles/10.3389/fimmu.2020.01648/full
25. Montazersaheb S, Hosseiniyan Khatibi SM, Hejazi MS, Tarhriz V, Farjami A, Ghasemian Sorbeni F, et al. COVID-19 infection: an overview on cytokine storm and related interventions. Virol J. 2022;19(1):92.
26. Tang Y, Liu J, Zhang D, Xu Z, Ji J, Wen C. Cytokine Storm in COVID-19: The Current Evidence and Treatment Strategies. Front Immunol [Internet]. 2020 [cited 2024 Oct 12];11. Available from: https://www.frontiersin.org/journals/immunology/articles/10.3389/fimmu.2020.01708/full
27. Saleh W, Hawky E, Halim GA, Ata F. Oral lichen planus after COVID-19, a case report. Ann Med Surg. 2021;(72):103051.
28. Scotto G, Fazio V, Massa S, Muzio LL, Spirito F. COVID-19 and oral lichen planus: between an "intriguing plot" and the "fata morgana effect". J Clin Med. 2023;12(14):4829.
29. Diab R, Araghi F, Gheisari M, Kani ZA, Moravvej H. Lichen planus and lichen planopilaris flare after COVID-19 vaccination. Dermatol Ther. 2022;35(3):e15283.
30. Gote V, Bolla PK, Kommineni N, Butreddy A, Nukala PK, Palakurthi SS, et al. A comprehensive review of mRNA vaccines. Int J Mol Sci. 2023 Jan;24(3):2700.
31. Deng S, Liang H, Chen P, Li Y, Li Z, Fan S, et al. Viral vector vaccine development and application during the COVID-19 pandemic. Microorganisms. 10(7):1450.
32. Vaccine Types | NIAID: National Institute of Allergy and Infectious Diseases [Internet]. 2019 [cited 2024 Oct 17]. Available from: https://www.niaid.nih.gov/research/vaccine-types
33. Trougakos IP, Terpos E, Alexopoulos H, Politou M, Paraskevis D, Scorilas A, et al. Adverse effects of COVID-19 mRNA vaccines: the spike hypothesis. Trends Mol Med. 2022;28(7):542.
34. Guimarães LE, Baker B, Perricone C, Shoenfeld Y. Vaccines, adjuvants and autoimmunity. Pharmacol Res. 2015;100:190.

35. Shim CH, Cho S, Shin YM, Choi JM. Emerging role of bystander T cell activation in autoimmune diseases. BMB Rep. 2022;55(2):57.
36. Arnold DL, Krishnamurthy K. Lichen Planus. In: StatPearls [Internet]. Treasure Island: StatPearls Publishing; 2024 [cited 2024 Oct 17]. Available from: http://www.ncbi.nlm.nih.gov/books/NBK526126/
37. Popa C, Sciuca AM, Onofrei BA, Toader S, Hritcu OMC, Colac CB, et al. Integrative approaches for the diagnosis and management of erosive oral lichen planus. Diagnostics. 2024;14(7):692.

6 The Effect of COVID-19 and Its Vaccination in Atopic Dermatitis Exacerbation

Aleksandra Ratkiewicz and Esraa M. AlEdani

6.1 Overview

Atopic dermatitis (AD), commonly known as eczema, is a chronic inflammatory skin condition characterized by pruritus (itching), erythema (redness), and a tendency toward a relapsing course. It often manifests in early childhood but can persist or emerge in adulthood. The pathogenesis of AD involves a complex interplay between genetic predisposition, immune system dysregulation, and environmental factors. It is associated with elevated serum immunoglobulin E (IgE) levels and a history of atopic diseases such as asthma and allergic rhinitis. The clinical presentation can vary widely, ranging from mild, localized patches to severe, widespread lesions, significantly impacting the quality of life of affected individuals [1].

Understanding the factors that exacerbate AD is crucial for effective management and improving patient outcomes. Exacerbating factors can include environmental triggers (such as allergens and pollutants), stress, infections, and hormonal changes. Identifying and mitigating these triggers can help reduce the frequency and severity of flares, leading to better disease control. Moreover, a comprehensive understanding of exacerbating factors can guide the development of targeted therapies and personalized treatment plans, ultimately enhancing patient care and reducing the burden of this chronic disease.

The COVID-19 pandemic, caused by the novel coronavirus SARS-CoV-2, has had a profound impact on global health since its emergence in late 2019. COVID-19 primarily manifests as a respiratory illness but can affect multiple organ systems, leading to a wide range of clinical presentations from asymptomatic cases to severe pneumonia and acute respiratory distress syndrome. The pandemic has necessitated unprecedented public health measures, including widespread social distancing, lockdowns, and the rapid development and deployment of vaccines. Vaccination has been a cornerstone in the fight against COVID-19, with several vaccines demonstrating high efficacy in preventing infection, severe disease, and death. The leading vaccines include mRNA-based vaccines (such as Pfizer-BioNTech and Moderna), vector-based vaccines (such as AstraZeneca and Johnson & Johnson), and inactivated vaccines (such as Sinovac and Sinopharm). These vaccines have been pivotal in curbing the spread of the virus and reducing the overall burden of the disease [2].

The intersection of COVID-19 and AD raises several important considerations. The pandemic has introduced new potential exacerbating fac-

A. Ratkiewicz (✉)
New York Institute of Technology College of Osteopathic Medicine (NYITCOM), Old Westbury, NY, USA
e-mail: aratkiew@nyit.edu

E. M. AlEdani
University of Basrah-Medical Faculty, Basrah, Iraq

E. M. AlEdani, H. Maibach (eds.), *COVID-19 Vaccination and Dermatological Diseases*, Updates in Clinical Dermatology, https://doi.org/10.1007/978-3-031-87791-9_6

tors for AD, such as increased stress, changes in lifestyle, and the use of personal protective equipment (PPE), which can irritate the skin. Additionally, there have been reports of cutaneous manifestations associated with COVID-19 infection, ranging from mild rashes to more severe inflammatory conditions. Understanding how COVID-19 directly or indirectly affects individuals with AD is crucial for developing effective management strategies during the pandemic.

Furthermore, the introduction of COVID-19 vaccinations has brought to light new questions regarding their safety and potential impact on individuals with AD. Vaccines, like any medical intervention, can have side effects, and there is a need to understand their implications for patients with pre-existing skin conditions. Some individuals with AD may be concerned about vaccine-related reactions, given their predisposition to inflammatory and allergic responses. Therefore, it is essential to evaluate the safety profile of COVID-19 vaccines in the context of AD and provide clear guidance to patients and healthcare providers [3].

In conclusion, atopic dermatitis is a prevalent and burdensome condition that can be significantly influenced by external factors, including infectious diseases like COVID-19 and its associated public health measures. Understanding the relationship between COVID-19, its vaccinations, and AD exacerbations is vital for optimizing patient care during and beyond the pandemic. This chapter aims to explore these interactions comprehensively, providing insights into the management of AD in the context of ongoing global health challenges [4].

6.2 Pathophysiology of Atopic Dermatitis

Genetic predisposition significantly contributes to the development of AD. Family history is a strong indicator, with a higher likelihood of AD in children whose parents have a history of atopic diseases, including asthma, allergic rhinitis, or AD itself. One of the most critical genetic factors identified is mutations in the FLG gene, which encodes filaggrin, a protein essential for the formation and maintenance of the skin barrier. Filaggrin aggregates keratin fibers in epidermal cells, facilitating the formation of the stratum corneum, the outermost layer of the skin. Mutations in the FLG gene result in a filaggrin deficiency, leading to a compromised skin barrier. This defect allows increased transepidermal water loss and greater penetration of allergens, irritants, and microbes, triggering inflammatory responses and predisposing individuals to AD [5].

Immune dysregulation is another cornerstone in the pathogenesis of AD. The immune response in AD is predominantly mediated by T-helper 2 (Th2) cells, which produce cytokines such as interleukin-4 (IL-4), interleukin-13 (IL-13), and interleukin-31 (IL-31). These cytokines promote IgE production by B cells, further fueling allergic inflammation. The Th2-skewed immune response also leads to a reduction in the production of antimicrobial peptides by keratinocytes, compromising the skin's ability to defend against microbial infections. During acute flares of AD, there is an increased expression of Th2 cytokines, whereas chronic AD lesions show a mixed Th2/Th1 cytokine profile, with elevated levels of interferon-gamma (IFN-γ) and interleukin-12 (IL-12). Additionally, recent studies have highlighted the role of other immune cells, such as Th22 and Th17 cells, in contributing to the chronicity and severity of AD [6].

Skin barrier dysfunction is a hallmark of AD and plays a pivotal role in its pathogenesis. The skin barrier consists of the stratum corneum and tight junctions between keratinocytes, which work together to maintain skin integrity and prevent the entry of harmful substances. In individuals with AD, the skin barrier is often compromised due to both genetic and environmental factors. Filaggrin deficiency, as mentioned earlier, is a primary genetic factor that disrupts the skin barrier. Additionally, decreased levels of ceramides, essential lipids in the stratum corneum, have been observed in AD patients, further weakening the barrier function [7].

Environmental factors, such as exposure to harsh soaps, detergents, and low humidity, can exacerbate skin barrier impairment. The compromised barrier allows allergens, microbes, and irritants to penetrate the skin more easily, triggering immune responses and inflammation. This increased permeability also leads to transepidermal water loss, contributing to the dry and scaly skin characteristic of AD. The ongoing inflammation and itching result in scratching, which further damages the skin barrier, creating a vicious cycle of barrier dysfunction and inflammation.

The pathophysiology of atopic dermatitis is a complex interplay of genetic predisposition, immune dysregulation, and skin barrier dysfunction. Understanding these interconnected mechanisms is crucial for developing effective treatments and management strategies for AD. Genetic factors, such as FLG mutations, highlight the importance of the skin barrier, while immune dysregulation underscores the role of inflammatory pathways in disease progression. Addressing both skin barrier integrity and immune modulation is essential in managing AD and improving the quality of life for affected individuals [8].

6.3 Impact of COVID-19 on Dermatological Conditions

The COVID-19 pandemic, caused by the novel coronavirus SARS-CoV-2, has profoundly impacted global health, affecting multiple organ systems, including the skin. Since the onset of the pandemic, numerous dermatological manifestations associated with COVID-19 have been reported. These manifestations range from common viral exanthems to unique presentations like "COVID toes." Understanding the relationship between COVID-19 and skin conditions, including atopic dermatitis (AD), is crucial for managing patients during this ongoing health crisis [9].

A comprehensive review of the literature reveals a diverse array of cutaneous manifestations associated with COVID-19. Early reports identified morbilliform eruptions, urticaria, and vesicular eruptions as common skin findings in COVID-19 patients. Subsequent studies expanded the spectrum of COVID-19-related dermatological conditions to include acral lesions, livedo reticularis, and purpuric rashes. Notably, "COVID toes" (chilblain-like lesions) became a well-recognized phenomenon, particularly in younger patients with mild or asymptomatic COVID-19. These lesions typically present as erythematous to violaceous papules on the toes and fingers and are thought to result from microvascular injury or an immune-mediated response to the virus [10].

The pathophysiology underlying these skin manifestations remains under investigation. Hypotheses include direct viral invasion of the skin, immune complex deposition, and thrombotic vasculopathy. Some cutaneous findings, such as morbilliform eruptions, may result from the body's systemic inflammatory response to the virus, while others, like livedo reticularis, may reflect underlying vascular injury and coagulopathy.

Specific to AD, several reports and studies have explored the impact of COVID-19 on this chronic inflammatory skin condition. AD patients, due to their compromised skin barrier and immune dysregulation, might be particularly vulnerable to changes induced by COVID-19 and related public health measures. A study by Gisondi et al. [5] investigated the effect of the pandemic on patients with pre-existing inflammatory skin diseases, including AD. The study found that a significant number of patients experienced disease exacerbations during the pandemic, which were attributed to multiple factors such as increased stress, changes in daily routines, and reduced access to dermatological care. Stress, in particular, is known to trigger or worsen AD by modulating immune responses and impairing skin barrier function. Additionally, case reports have documented AD exacerbations in COVID-19 patients. For instance, a report by Piccolo et al. [6] described a patient with well-controlled AD who experienced a severe flare following a COVID-19 infection. The exacerbation was characterized by widespread eczematous lesions and intense pruritus, necessitating systemic corticosteroids for management. The authors hypothesized that the systemic inflammatory response induced by SARS-CoV-2 infection, combined with the stress and anxiety associated with the disease, contributed to the AD flare [11].

Another consideration is the impact of personal protective equipment (PPE) on AD patients. Prolonged use of masks and gloves, essential for preventing the spread of COVID-19, can aggravate AD by causing friction, occlusion, and sweating, leading to irritant contact dermatitis. This can be particularly challenging for healthcare workers with pre-existing AD, as they are required to wear PPE for extended periods [12].

In conclusion, the COVID-19 pandemic has significantly impacted dermatological conditions, including atopic dermatitis. The diverse cutaneous manifestations associated with COVID-19 highlight the virus's potential to affect the skin through various mechanisms. For AD patients, the pandemic has introduced new challenges, including increased stress, reduced access to care, and the adverse effects of PPE. Understanding these factors is crucial for managing AD exacerbations during the pandemic and ensuring optimal patient care. As the pandemic continues, further research is needed to elucidate the long-term effects of COVID-19 on dermatological conditions and to develop strategies to mitigate these impacts [13].

6.4 Mechanisms of Exacerbation in Atopic Dermatitis

The COVID-19 pandemic has had a multifaceted impact on individuals with atopic dermatitis (AD), leading to exacerbations through several mechanisms. These include the stress and psychological impact of the pandemic, the immune response to viral infections, and the disruption of routine care. Understanding these mechanisms is essential for developing effective strategies to manage AD during such unprecedented times.

The psychological burden imposed by the COVID-19 pandemic has been significant, contributing to increased stress levels across populations. For individuals with AD, stress is a well-known trigger that can exacerbate their condition. The pandemic has introduced various stressors, including fear of infection, social isolation, financial uncertainties, and changes in daily routines. Chronic stress can impair skin barrier function, promote inflammatory pathways, and trigger itch-scratch cycles, all of which can lead to worsening of AD symptoms. Studies have shown that stress can influence the hypothalamic-pituitary-adrenal (HPA) axis, resulting in the release of cortisol and other stress hormones that can negatively impact skin health. Additionally, stress-induced neuropeptides, such as substance P and calcitonin gene-related peptide (CGRP), can directly contribute to skin inflammation and itch [14].

The immune response to viral infections, including SARS-CoV-2, can significantly impact individuals with AD. Viral infections often induce a systemic inflammatory response, which can exacerbate underlying inflammatory conditions like AD. The immune dysregulation inherent in AD patients, characterized by a Th2-skewed response, can interact with the body's response to viral infections, leading to heightened inflammatory activity. For instance, SARS-CoV-2 infection triggers the release of a plethora of cytokines, including interleukin-6 (IL-6) and tumor necrosis factor-alpha (TNF-α), which can amplify skin inflammation in AD patients. Additionally, the skin manifestations associated with COVID-19, such as viral exanthems or "COVID toes," might further complicate the clinical picture of AD, making it more challenging to manage the disease effectively [15].

The COVID-19 pandemic has significantly disrupted routine healthcare services, impacting the management of chronic conditions such as AD. Lockdowns, social distancing measures, and the reallocation of healthcare resources have led to reduced access to dermatological care. Regular follow-ups, in-person consultations, and elective procedures have been postponed or canceled, leading to gaps in patient care. This disruption can result in inadequate disease monitoring, delayed treatment adjustments, and increased disease flares. Moreover, the pandemic has affected the availability and affordability of medications, which are crucial for maintaining AD control. Many patients have faced challenges in obtaining their prescribed treatments, leading to suboptimal disease management [16].

The use of personal protective equipment (PPE) has been essential for preventing the spread of COVID-19 but has also posed challenges for AD patients. Prolonged use of masks and gloves can cause friction, occlusion, and sweating, leading to irritant contact dermatitis. For healthcare workers with pre-existing AD, the mandatory use of PPE can exacerbate their condition, causing discomfort and worsening skin symptoms. The increased hand hygiene practices, involving frequent washing and the use of alcohol-based sanitizers, can further irritate the skin and disrupt the skin barrier, contributing to AD flares.

The exacerbation of atopic dermatitis during the COVID-19 pandemic can be attributed to multiple interconnected mechanisms, including the stress and psychological impact of the pandemic, the immune response to viral infections, and the disruption of routine care. Understanding these factors is crucial for healthcare providers to develop comprehensive management strategies for AD patients in the context of the ongoing pandemic. Addressing stress, ensuring continuity of care, and mitigating the adverse effects of PPE use are essential components of managing AD exacerbations during this challenging time. As the pandemic continues, further research is needed to explore the long-term impacts on AD and to refine management approaches to improve patient outcomes [17].

6.5 The Role of COVID-19 Vaccinations in Atopic Dermatitis

The COVID-19 pandemic has necessitated the rapid development and deployment of vaccines to mitigate the spread of SARS-CoV-2 and reduce morbidity and mortality. These vaccines have been crucial in controlling the pandemic, but their impact on individuals with pre-existing conditions, such as atopic dermatitis (AD), warrants careful consideration. This section explores the different types of COVID-19 vaccines, their mechanisms, reported cases of vaccine-associated dermatological reactions, and insights from clinical trials and observational studies regarding their effects on AD [18].

Several COVID-19 vaccines have been developed, each employing different technologies and mechanisms to elicit an immune response. The primary types include mRNA vaccines, viral vector vaccines, protein subunit vaccines, and inactivated vaccines (Table 6.1).

Since the rollout of COVID-19 vaccines, various dermatological reactions have been reported. These reactions range from mild and transient to more severe and persistent, although they are generally rare. Commonly reported reactions include local injection site reactions, urticaria (hives), and morbilliform (measles-like) rashes. Local reactions at the injection site, such as pain, redness, and swelling, are the most common dermatological side effects. These typically resolve within a few days without intervention. Urticaria, or hives, characterized by itchy, raised welts on the skin, has been reported following vaccination. These reactions can occur within minutes to hours post-vaccination and are usually self-limiting. Morbilliform rashes, presenting as widespread, erythematous macules and papules, have also been observed. These rashes typically appear within a week of vaccination and resolve spontaneously. More severe reactions, such as erythema multiforme, a hypersensitivity reaction presenting with target-like lesions, have been reported but are exceedingly rare. There have also been isolated reports of psoriasis flares and new-onset inflammatory skin conditions following vaccination [19].

Clinical trials and observational studies provide critical insights into the safety and efficacy of COVID-19 vaccines, particularly in individuals with pre-existing conditions like AD. Initial clinical trials of COVID-19 vaccines primarily focused on the general population, including individuals with chronic diseases. However, specific data on patients with AD were limited. These trials demonstrated high efficacy of the vaccines in preventing COVID-19, with a favorable safety profile. Common adverse events were

Table 6.1 Table of vaccine types, examples of market vaccines, and mechanisms of action

Vaccine type	Vaccine example	Description
mRNA	Pfizer-BioNTech (Comirnaty) and Moderna (Spikevax) vaccines	These vaccines use lipid nanoparticles to deliver a synthetic mRNA encoding the SARS-CoV-2 spike protein into host cells. The host cells then produce the spike protein, which prompts an immune response, including the production of neutralizing antibodies and activation of T-cells
Viral Vector	AstraZeneca (Vaxzevria) and Johnson & Johnson (Janssen) vaccines	These vaccines use adenoviral vectors to deliver the gene for the SARS-CoV-2 spike protein. These vectors are modified viruses that cannot replicate but can induce an immune response by presenting the spike protein to the immune system
Protein Subunit	Novavax vaccine	These vaccines use purified pieces of the SARS-CoV-2 spike protein (subunits) to stimulate an immune response without using live virus components. These vaccines often include adjuvants to enhance the immune response
Inactivated	Sinovac (CoronaVac) and Sinopharm vaccines	These vaccines use inactivated (killed) versions of the SARS-CoV-2 virus. These vaccines cannot cause disease but can stimulate an immune response through the presentation of viral proteins

mostly mild to moderate, including local and systemic reactions such as fever, fatigue, and myalgia. Subsequent observational studies have provided more detailed information on the impact of COVID-19 vaccines on patients with AD. A study investigating the dermatological reactions to COVID-19 vaccines in patients with various skin conditions, including AD, found that while some patients with AD reported mild flares following vaccination, these were generally manageable with standard AD treatments and did not necessitate discontinuation of the vaccine series. Case reports and series have documented specific instances of AD exacerbations following COVID-19 vaccination. These exacerbations were generally mild to moderate and responded well to topical corticosteroids and moisturizers. Transient immune activation induced by the vaccines might trigger AD flares in susceptible individuals but these reactions should not deter patients from getting vaccinated [20].

The exact mechanisms by which COVID-19 vaccines may exacerbate AD are not fully understood but are likely multifactorial. Vaccines induce a robust immune response, which can include the activation of T-helper cells and the release of various cytokines. In individuals with AD, whose immune systems are already dysregulated, this heightened immune activity could potentially trigger or worsen inflammatory skin responses. Additionally, the stress and anxiety associated with vaccination, particularly in individuals with a history of severe allergic reactions, could contribute to AD exacerbations through psychoneuroimmunological pathways.

COVID-19 vaccines play a crucial role in controlling the pandemic and are generally safe for individuals with atopic dermatitis. While there have been reports of dermatological reactions and AD exacerbations following vaccination, these incidents are relatively rare and typically mild. The benefits of vaccination in preventing severe COVID-19 far outweigh the risks of potential skin reactions. Clinical trials and observational studies support the safety and efficacy of these vaccines, even in populations with pre-existing skin conditions. Healthcare providers should continue to monitor patients with AD closely and provide appropriate management for any vaccine-related skin reactions, ensuring that these patients receive the full benefits of COVID-19 vaccination while maintaining control of their chronic skin condition. Further research is needed to elucidate the precise mechanisms behind vaccine-associated AD exacerbations and to develop strategies to mitigate these effects, thereby enhancing patient care during and beyond the pandemic [21].

6.6 Management Strategies for Atopic Dermatitis During the Pandemic

The COVID-19 pandemic has necessitated adaptations in the management of chronic conditions such as atopic dermatitis (AD). Given the challenges posed by the pandemic, effective management strategies are crucial to maintaining disease control and ensuring patient well-being. Key strategies include the importance of telemedicine, modification of treatment plans, and psychological support for patients [22].

Telemedicine has emerged as a vital tool for managing atopic dermatitis during the pandemic. The necessity for social distancing and the risk of COVID-19 exposure in healthcare settings have made telemedicine an essential service. Teledermatology allows for remote consultation, diagnosis, and treatment, enabling continuous care without requiring patients to leave their homes. It is particularly beneficial for patients with AD, who require regular monitoring and frequent adjustments to their treatment plans. Through telemedicine, dermatologists can evaluate the severity of AD, assess treatment efficacy, and provide timely interventions. High-quality video consultations and digital photography enable clinicians to examine skin lesions accurately. Additionally, telemedicine platforms often include secure messaging, allowing patients to report new symptoms, seek advice, and receive prescriptions promptly. This continuity of care helps prevent disease exacerbations and ensures that patients adhere to their treatment regimens [23].

The pandemic has prompted a reevaluation and modification of treatment plans for patients with atopic dermatitis. Regular in-person visits and procedures may be limited, so treatment plans must be flexible and adaptable to changing circumstances. Dermatologists are increasingly prescribing treatments that are convenient for home use and have a favorable safety profile to minimize the need for frequent office visits. For mild to moderate AD, topical therapies such as corticosteroids, calcineurin inhibitors, and moisturizers remain the mainstay of treatment. Dermatologists might also recommend over-the-counter emollients to maintain skin hydration and barrier function. For patients with more severe AD, systemic treatments such as biologics (e.g., dupilumab) can be administered at home, reducing the need for in-clinic infusions or injections [24].

Moreover, the pandemic has highlighted the importance of patient education. Patients are being empowered with knowledge about proper skincare routines, trigger avoidance, and early signs of exacerbation. Educated patients are better equipped to manage their condition independently, which is particularly valuable when access to healthcare services is limited.

The psychological impact of the COVID-19 pandemic on patients with atopic dermatitis cannot be overstated. AD is often exacerbated by stress, and the pandemic has introduced numerous stressors, including fear of infection, social isolation, financial concerns, and disruptions to daily life. Psychological support is therefore a critical component of comprehensive AD management. Healthcare providers should actively screen for anxiety, depression, and other mental health issues in their AD patients. Providing psychological support can include referring patients to mental health professionals, offering counseling services, and encouraging participation in support groups. Cognitive-behavioral therapy (CBT) has been shown to be particularly effective in helping patients manage stress and cope with chronic disease. Additionally, dermatologists can support their patients by fostering a reassuring and empathetic communication style during consultations. Understanding and addressing the psychological burdens of AD can improve patient outcomes and adherence to treatment plans. Online support communities and resources can also provide a sense of connection and shared experience for patients feeling isolated due to their condition [25].

Managing atopic dermatitis during the COVID-19 pandemic requires a multifaceted approach that adapts to the unique challenges presented by the current healthcare landscape. Telemedicine offers a practical solution for continuous care, while flexible treatment plans ensure that patients can manage their condition effectively at home. Psychological support addresses the mental health challenges exacerbated by the pandemic, helping patients maintain both physical and emotional well-being. By integrating these strategies, healthcare providers can ensure comprehensive and effective management of atopic dermatitis, even in the midst of a global health crisis [26].

6.7 Conclusion

The COVID-19 pandemic has presented significant challenges for individuals with atopic dermatitis (AD), impacting the pathophysiology, management, and overall disease burden of this chronic condition. This chapter has explored the intricate relationship between COVID-19, its vaccinations, and the exacerbations of AD, providing a comprehensive understanding of the multifaceted effects of the pandemic on dermatological health [27].

The emergence of COVID-19 has had a profound impact on dermatological conditions, including AD. Various skin manifestations associated with COVID-19, such as morbilliform eruptions and "COVID toes," highlight the virus's capacity to affect the skin. AD patients have reported disease exacerbations during the pandemic, influenced by increased stress, reduced access to care, and changes in daily routines. The systemic inflammatory response to SARS-CoV-2 infection can further aggravate underlying dermatological conditions, necessitating careful management and monitoring [28].

The exacerbation of AD during the pandemic can be attributed to several mechanisms. The psychological impact of the pandemic, including increased stress and anxiety, plays a significant role in triggering AD flares. Stress can impair skin barrier function and modulate immune responses, leading to worsening symptoms. Additionally, the immune response to viral infections, such as SARS-CoV-2, can amplify skin inflammation in AD patients. The disruption of routine care due to lockdowns and healthcare system strains has also contributed to increased disease activity, as patients face challenges in accessing necessary treatments and follow-up appointments [29].

COVID-19 vaccinations have been instrumental in controlling the pandemic, but their impact on AD warrants consideration. Different vaccine types, including mRNA, viral vector, protein subunit, and inactivated vaccines, have been developed, each with unique mechanisms of action. While most dermatological reactions to vaccines are mild and transient, there have been reports of urticaria, morbilliform rashes, and rare severe reactions. Clinical trials and observational studies have generally shown that vaccines are safe for individuals with AD, with only a small percentage experiencing exacerbations. The benefits of vaccination in preventing severe COVID-19 outweigh the risks of potential skin reactions.

Effective management of AD during the pandemic involves adapting to the new challenges posed by COVID-19. Telemedicine has emerged as a crucial tool, enabling continuous care and reducing the risk of exposure to the virus. Dermatologists can assess and manage AD remotely, ensuring timely interventions and maintaining treatment adherence. Modifying treatment plans to include home-administered therapies and educating patients about proper skincare routines have been essential in minimizing disease flares. Additionally, providing psychological support is critical, as stress and anxiety can exacerbate AD. Screening for mental health issues and offering counseling or cognitive-behavioral therapy can significantly improve patient outcomes [30].

In summary, the COVID-19 pandemic has intricately affected atopic dermatitis through various mechanisms, including stress, immune response, and healthcare disruptions. Understanding the pathophysiology of AD and the impact of the pandemic on dermatological conditions is crucial for effective management. COVID-19 vaccinations, while generally safe, require careful consideration in AD patients, with vigilant monitoring for potential exacerbations. Telemedicine, flexible treatment plans, and psychological support are essential strategies for managing AD during these challenging times. As the pandemic continues to evolve, ongoing research and adaptation of management approaches will be necessary to ensure optimal care for individuals with atopic dermatitis [31].

References

1. Martora F, Battista T, Ruggiero A, Scalvenzi M, Villani A, Megna M, Potestio L. The impact of COVID-19 vaccination on inflammatory skin disorders and other cutaneous diseases: a review of the published literature. Viruses. 2023;15:1423. https://doi.org/10.3390/v15071423.
2. Marko M, Pawliczak R. Can we safely use systemic treatment in atopic dermatitis during the COVID-19 pandemic? Overview of selected conventional and biologic systemic therapies. Expert Rev Clin Immunol. 2021;17(6):619–27. https://doi.org/10.1080/1744666X.2021.1919511.
3. Schuler CF, Billi AC, Maverakis E, Tsoi LC, Gudjonsson JE, Novel insights into atopic dermatitis. J Allergy Clin Immunol. 2023; 151(5):1145–1154.https://doi.org/10.1016/j.jaci.2022.10.023. ISSN 0091-6749
4. Mahdiabadi S, Rajabi F, Tavakolpour S, Rezaei N. Immunological aspects of COVID-19-related skin manifestations: revisiting pathogenic mechanism in the light of new evidence. Dermatol Ther. 2022;35(10):e15758. https://doi.org/10.1111/dth.15758.
5. Gisondi P, Di Leo S, Bellinato F, et al. Time of onset of selected skin lesions associated with COVID-19: a systematic review. Dermatol Ther (Heidelb). 2021;11:695–705. https://doi.org/10.1007/s13555-021-00526-8.
6. Piccolo V, Neri I, Filippeschi C, Oranges T, Argenziano G, Battarra VC, Berti S, Manunza F, Fortina AB, Di Lernia V, Boccaletti V, De Bernardis G, Brunetti B, Mazzatenta C, Bassi A. Chilblain-like lesions during COVID-19 epidemic: a preliminary study on 63 patients. J Eur Acad Dermatol Venereol. 2020;34(7):e291–3. https://doi.org/10.1111/jdv.16526. Epub 2020 May 15. PMID: 32330334; PMCID: PMC7267498.
7. Neri I, Galli E, Baiardini I, Picozza M, Rossi AB, Matruglio P, et al. Implications of atopic dermatitis on the quality of life of 6–11 years old children and caregivers (PEDI-BURDEN). J Asthma Allergy. 2023;16:383–96. https://doi.org/10.2147/JAA.S404350.
8. El-Qushayri AE, Mahmoud MA, Salman S, Sarsik S, Nardone B. Dupilumab therapy in atopic dermatitis is safe during COVID-19 infection era: a systematic review and meta-analysis of 1611 patients. Dermatol Ther. 2022;35(6):e15476.
9. Abdali, Selli et al. Occupational dermatoses related to personal protective equipment used during the COVID-19 pandemic. Dermatol Clinics;39(4):555–68.
10. Thyssen JP, Vestergaard C, Barbarot S, de Bruin-Weller MS, Bieber T, Taieb A, Seneschal J, Cork MJ, Paul C, Flohr C, Weidinger S, Trzeciak M, Werfel T, Heratizadeh A, Darsow U, Simon D, Torrelo A, Chernyshov PV, Stalder J-F, Gelmetti C, Szalai Z, Svensson Å, von Kobyletzki LB, De Raeve L, Fölster-Holst R, Christen-Zaech S, Hijnen DJ, Gieler U, Gutermuth J, Bangert C, Spuls PI, Kunz B, Ring J, Wollenberg A, Deleuran M. European Task Force on Atopic Dermatitis: position on vaccination of adult patients with atopic dermatitis against COVID-19 (SARS-CoV-2) being treated with systemic medication and biologics. J Eur Acad Dermatol Venereol. 2021;35:e308–11. https://doi.org/10.1111/jdv.17167.
11. Leasure AC, Cowper SE, McNiff J, Cohen JM. Generalized eczematous reactions to the Pfizer-BioNTech COVID-19 vaccine. J Eur Acad Dermatol Venereol. 2021;35(11):e716–7. https://doi.org/10.1111/jdv.17494. Epub 2021 Jul 26. PMID: 34236729; PMCID: PMC8447468.
12. Bettini E, Locci M. SARS-CoV-2 mRNA vaccines: immunological mechanism and beyond. Vaccine. 2021;9(2):147. https://doi.org/10.3390/vaccines9020147.
13. Lamprinou M, Sachinidis A, Stamoula E, et al. COVID-19 vaccines adverse events: potential molecular mechanisms. Immunol Res. 2023;71:356–72. https://doi.org/10.1007/s12026-023-09357-5.
14. McMahon DE, Amerson E, Rosenbach M, Lipoff JB, Moustafa D, Tyagi A, et al. Cutaneous reactions reported after Moderna and Pfizer COVID-19 vaccination: a registry-based study of 414 cases. J Am Acad Dermatol. 2021;85(1):46–55.
15. Mahapatra S, Nagpal R, Marya CM, Taneja P, Kataria S. Adverse events occurring post-covid-19 vaccination among healthcare professionals—a mixed method study. Int Immunopharmacol. 2021;100:108136.
16. Judd A, Samarakoon U, Wolfson AR, Banerji A, Freeman EE, Blumenthal KG. Urticaria after COVID-19 vaccination and vaccine hesitancy. J Allergy Clin Immunol Pract. 2023;11(3):958.
17. Jedlowski PM, Jedlowski MF. Morbilliform rash after administration of Pfizer-BioNTech COVID-19 mRNA vaccine. Dermatol Online J. 2021;27(1).
18. Novak N, Tordesillas L, Cabanillas B. Adverse rare events to vaccines for COVID-19: from hypersensitivity reactions to thrombosis and thrombocytopenia. Int Rev Immunol. 2022;41(4):438–47.
19. Grieco T, Maddalena P, Sernicola A, Muharremi R, Basili S, Alvaro D, et al. Cutaneous adverse reactions after COVID-19 vaccines in a cohort of 2740 Italian subjects: an observational study. Dermatol Ther. 2021;34(6):e15153.
20. Al Khames Aga QA, Alkhaffaf WH, Hatem TH, Nassir KF, Batineh Y, Dahham AT, et al. Safety of COVID-19 vaccines. J Med Virol. 2021;93(12):6588–94.
21. Niebel D, Novak N, Wilhelmi J, Ziob J, Wilsmann-Theis D, Bieber T, et al. Cutaneous adverse reac-

tions to COVID-19 vaccines: insights from an immuno-dermatological perspective. Vaccine. 2021;9(9):944.
22. Magro C, Crowson AN, Franks L, Schaffer PR, Whelan P, Nuovo G. The histologic and molecular correlates of COVID-19 vaccine-induced changes in the skin. Clin Dermatol. 2021;39(6):966–84.
23. Marasca C, Annunziata MC, Camela E, Di Guida A, Fornaro L, Megna M, et al. Teledermatology and inflammatory skin conditions during COVID-19 era: new perspectives and applications. J Clin Med. 2022;11(6):1511.
24. Loh CH, Tam SYC, Oh CC. Teledermatology in the COVID-19 pandemic: a systematic review. JAAD Int. 2021;5:54–64.
25. Ibrahim AE, Magdy M, Khalaf EM, Mostafa A, Arafa A. Teledermatology in the time of COVID-19. Int J Clin Pract. 2021;75(12):e15000.
26. Fishbein AB, Silverberg JI, Wilson EJ, Ong PY. Update on atopic dermatitis: diagnosis, severity assessment, and treatment selection. J Allergy Clin Immunol Pract. 2020;8(1):91–101.
27. Patel A, Jafferany M. Multidisciplinary and holistic models of care for patients with dermatologic disease and psychosocial comorbidity: a systematic review. JAMA Dermatol. 2020;156(6):686–94.
28. Nobari NN, Goodarzi A. Patients with specific skin disorders who are affected by COVID-19: what do experiences say about management strategies? A systematic review. Dermatol Ther. 2020;33(6):e13867.
29. Wollina U. Challenges of COVID-19 pandemic for dermatology. Dermatol Ther. 2020;33(5):e13430.
30. Beiu C, Mihai M, Popa L, Cima L, Popescu MN. Frequent hand washing for COVID-19 prevention can cause hand dermatitis: management tips. Cureus. 2020;12(4).
31. Fan R, Leasure AC, Damsky W, Cohen JM. Association between atopic dermatitis and COVID-19 infection: a case-control study in the All of Us research program. JAAD Int. 2022;6:77–81.

Effects of COVID-19 and Its Vaccination on Bullous Pemphigoid

7

Jhanvi Sawlani and Esraa M. AlEdani

7.1 Introduction

7.1.1 Overview of Bullous Pemphigoid

Bullous Pemphigoid is the most common type of autoimmune bullous dermatosis [1]. It is a chronic condition characterised by the formation of large, tense, fluid-filled blisters on the skin, commonly seen in the elderly.

It is driven by autoantibodies targeting the Bullous Pemphigoid180 (collagen type XVII) and Bullous Pemphigoid230 proteins in the skin's basement membrane at the subepidermal level. While a variety of genetic, environmental, and age-related factors contribute to the disease's onset and progression, the exact mechanisms remain the subject of ongoing research. However, a thorough understanding of these causes is essential for effective management and treatment of the condition (Fig. 7.1).

According to severity, management of Bullous Pemphigoid typically includes alone or a combination of topical and/or systemic steroids, immunosuppressants as well as adjuncts like antihistamines [2].

The emergence of the COVID-19 pandemic and the subsequent roll-out of COVID-19 vaccines have had profound effects on healthcare systems worldwide, including on the diagnosis and management of autoimmune conditions like Bullous Pemphigoid.

The onset of Bullous Pemphigoid-like cutaneous manifestations post vaccine administration has been seen with vaccines against tetanus, poliomyelitis, diphtheria, influenza, pneumococcus, meningococcus, hepatitis B and rabies [3]. Similar cutaneous manifestations along with others have been reported following COVID-19 vaccination [4–6].

While many new onset dermatological manifestations have been observed post Covid 19 infection, bullous pemphigoid remains one of the less common conditions reported. On the other hand, the COVID 19 vaccine seems to have some impact on new onset Bullous Pemphigoid as well as Bullous Pemphigoid flares that are yet to be further researched.

This chapter explores, based on information available so far, the impact of the COVID-19 pandemic and its vaccination on the incidence, progression, and management of bullous pemphigoid.

J. Sawlani (✉)
Department of Endocrinology, University Hospitals Birmingham, Birmingham, UK

E. M. AlEdani
University of Basrah-Medical Faculty, Basrah, Iraq

E. M. AlEdani, H. Maibach (eds.), *COVID-19 Vaccination and Dermatological Diseases*, Updates in Clinical Dermatology, https://doi.org/10.1007/978-3-031-87791-9_7

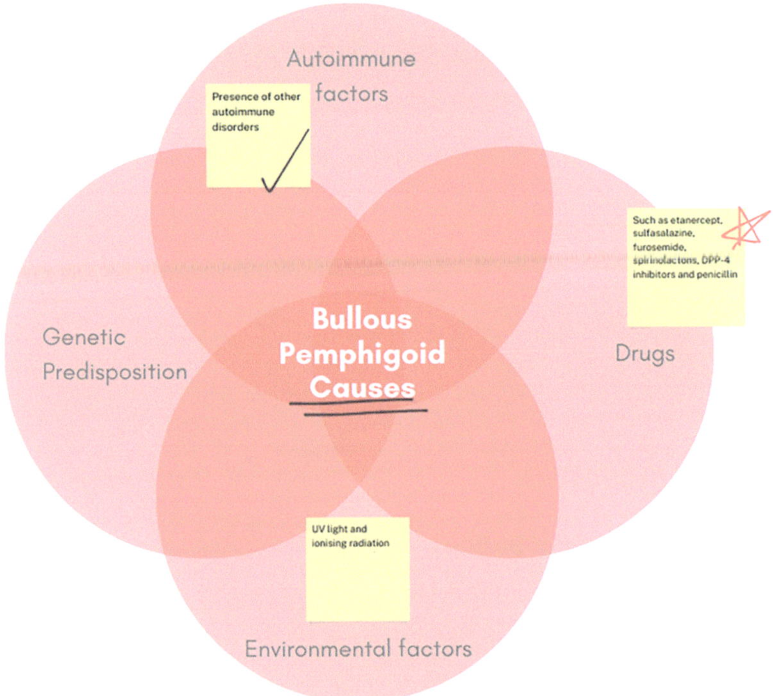

Fig. 7.1 Bullous Pemphigoid causes

7.1.2 Clinical Presentation of BP

- Commonly starts with complaints of itchy skin for weeks or months before blisters appear [7]
- Large, tense, fluid-filled blisters over normal or erythematous skin, that don't easily rupture when touched, often along creases or folds in the skin (Fig. 7.2) [7, 8]
- Can be clear fluid or blood stained
- Eczema or a hive-like rash
- Blisters can be generalised throughout the body and form anywhere, especially on the trunk, proximal limbs and flexures.
- Localised bullous pemphigoid is less common, and is usually limited to the lower extremities.

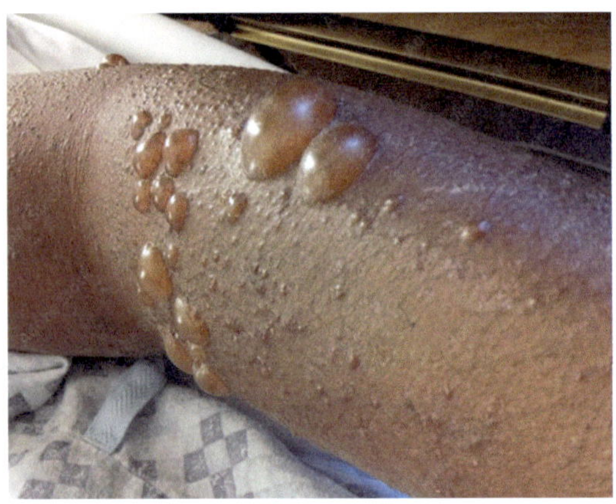

Fig. 7.2 Morphology of blisters in Bullous Pemphigoid

7.1.3 Risk Factors Associated with Bullous Pemphigoid Include

- Psoriasis
- Lichen planus
- Diabetes
- Ulcerative colitis
- Multiple sclerosis
- Neurological disorders, including dementia, Parkinson's disease, stroke, epilepsy, Shy-Drager syndrome, amyotrophic lateral sclerosis and multiple sclerosis– The association of neurological diseases with bullous pemphigoid is attributed to the presence of collagen type XVII within the hemidesmosomes of the central nervous system and skin [9].

- Autoimmune disorders like rheumatoid arthritis and lupus
- Certain medications used to treat autoimmune disorders

7.1.4 Pathophysiology of BP

Bullous pemphigoid is the result of an attack on the basement membrane of the epidermis mainly by IgG +/− IgE immunoglobulins and activated T lymphocytes [2].

The target is the protein Bullous Pemphigoid180 (also called Type XVII collagen), or less frequently Bullous Pemphigoid230 (a plakin). They are associated with the hemidesmosomes, structures that ensure the epidermal keratinocyte cells stick to the dermis to make a leak-proof seal.

The binding of the autoantibodies to the proteins and release of cytokines from the T cells lead to complement activation, recruitment of neutrophils (acute inflammatory cells) and the release of proteolytic enzymes. These destroy the hemidesmosomes and cause the formation of subepidermal blisters (Fig. 7.3).

7.1.5 Diagnosis of BP (Fig. 7.4)

Bloods Tests—Indirect Immunofluorescence

- **Skin antibodies include** both pemphigoid (skin basement membrane) and pemphigus (skin desmosome) antibodies. In bullous pemphigoid, circulating pemphigoid antibodies are present in approximately 75% of patients [10]

Skin Biopsies—Histology and Direct Immunofluorescence

- **Two biopsies from the skin are required**
  - **For histology:** An **intact blister** should be excised and sent
  - For DIF (**direct immunofluorescence**) **:**A second tissue sample of **skin within two cm of the blister**
  - **Findings that confirm bullous pemphigoid**
    - **Histologically** - the **blister is subepidermal** and contains fibrin and large

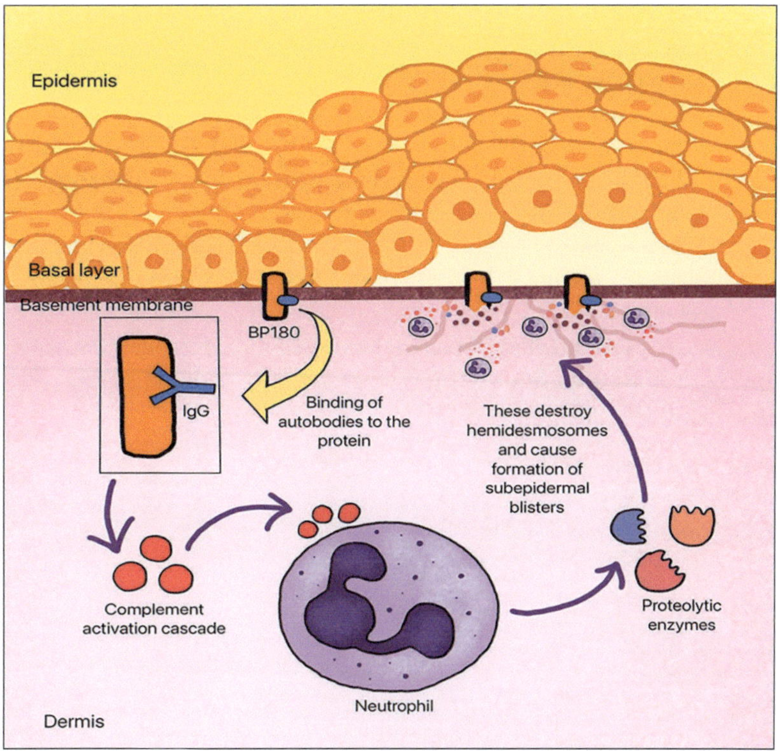

Fig. 7.3 Autoantibodies (IgG/IgE) bind to BP180/BP230 proteins in hemidesmosomes—T lymphocytes release cytokines—Cytokines activate and attract neutrophils to the basement membrane zone—Neutrophils release proteolytic enzymes—Proteolytic enzymes degrade hemidesmosomes—subepidermal blister forms due to the separation of the epidermis from the dermis

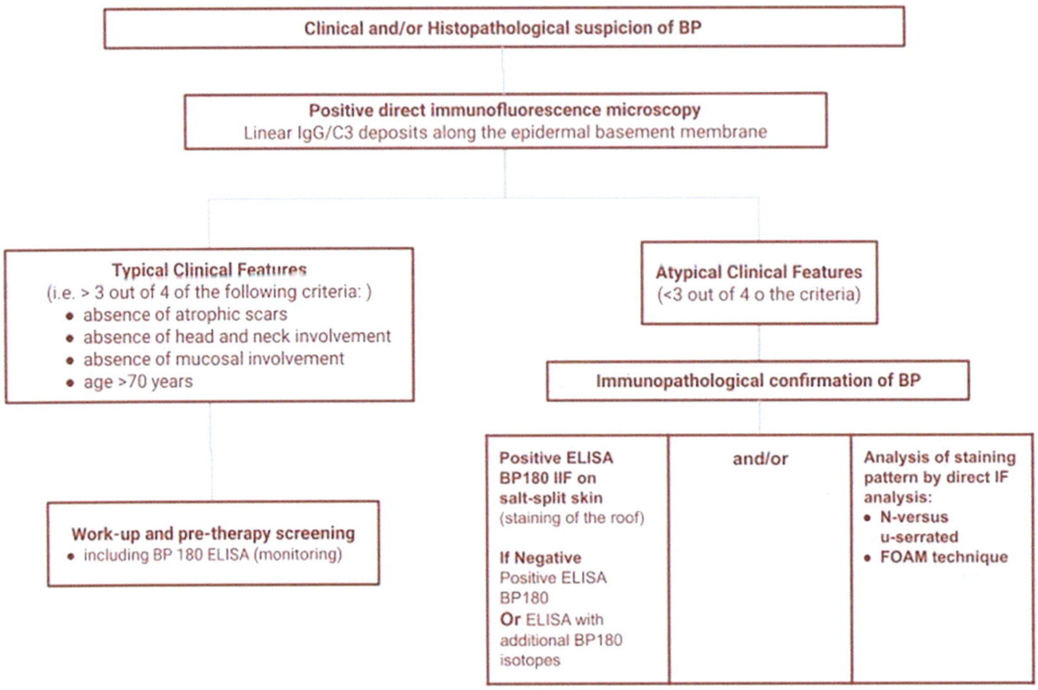

Fig. 7.4 Diagnostic algorithm for Bullous Pemphigoid

numbers of inflammatory cells including eosinophils, which may be very dense in areas and form small abscesses in the superficial dermis. The epidermis should be intact

- **DIF** shows linear deposition of **IgG (most often IgG4 subtype) and C3 to BP180 and BP230 along the basement membrane**. IgA and IgM deposition may be noted.

- **Special testing :** Salt-split skin technique:
  - Helps differentiate from epidermolysis bullosa acquisita
  - In BP: IgG appears on blister roof (epidermal side)
  - In EBA: IgG appears on blister floor (dermal side) [11]

7.1.6 Management of BP—Stepwise Approach (Fig. 7.5)

General Measures

1. Urgent secondary care referral needed for most patients
2. Hospital admission may be required for extensive blistering

Fig. 7.5 Stepwise management of Bullous Pemphigoid

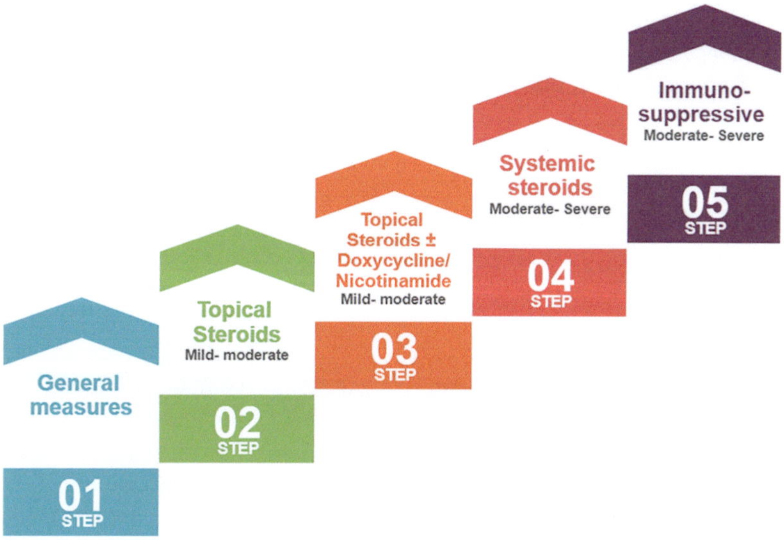

3. Basic care includes:
   - Wound management
   - Infection prevention using antiseptic solutions (e.g., Dermol 500 lotion)
   - Primary care management suitable only for limited cases

Localised Disease: Super-Potent Topical Steroids

- Dermovate® cream (clobetasol) is a very effective treatment for localised disease. In more severe disease, it can be used twice a day
- side effects are very much less compared to systemic steroids

Localised Mild-Moderate: Other Treatments

- *Doxycycline 100 mg BD*
- There is also some evidence for nicotinamide

Moderate- Severe: Systemic Steroids

- Systemic steroids are the **mainstay of treatment**.

The initial dose is as follows:

- 20 mg/day in localised-mild disease
- 40 mg/day in moderate disease
- 50–70 mg/day in severe disease

Tapering schedule:

- Initial reduction to 15–20 mg/day over weeks
- Below 10 mg/day: reduce by 1 mg/month
- Increase dose if blisters recur, then restart gradual reduction

Required precautions for adverse effects:

- Gastric protection (PPI)
- Osteoporosis prevention
- Regular Blood pressure monitoring
- Regular Blood glucose monitoring

Moderate- Severe: Other Treatments

- Immunosuppressive drugs such as methotrexate and mycophenolate mofetil are generally

only considered if the steroid dose cannot be reduced to an acceptable level
- The role of biologic therapies remains unclear

7.1.7 Prognosis

Prognosis varies significantly based on disease severity:

Severe/Generalised Disease:
- Typical duration: 3–6 years
- Poor prognostic indicators:
  - Widespread disease involvement
  - Low albumin levels
  - Need for high-dose steroid therapy
- Can be potentially fatal

Localised Disease
- Generally favourable outlook
- Better treatment response
- Lower risk of complications

7.1.8 Complications

- Skin infections—Bacterial skin infections, including *Staphylococcal* and *Streptococcal* infections as well as Viral infections, such as those caused by *Herpes simplex*, *Varicella*, or *Herpes zoster*
- Sepsis
- Dehydration
- Morbidity and mortality (severe cases and elderly)
- **Medication-Related Risks:** Osteoporosis, Cataracts

7.2 Impact of COVID-19 on Bullous Pemphigoid

The SARS-CoV-2 virus triggered a worldwide health crisis leading to the COVID-19 pandemic starting in late 2019 [13]. Initial COVID-19 infections ranged from showing no symptoms to causing life-threatening complications. Common early symptoms included fever, breathing difficulties, and cough, with some patients developing severe lung inflammation and respiratory failure (ARDS). In the most critical cases, multiple organ failure.

A significant medical challenge emerged as many patients developed ongoing health issues after their initial recovery, termed "long COVID" or PASC [14]. These persistent problems include extreme tiredness, breathing difficulties, heart complications, and cognitive issues like mental fogginess. The virus has also been linked to immune system disruptions, potentially triggering new autoimmune conditions or worsening existing ones. One example is multisystem inflammatory syndrome (MIS), showcasing how COVID-19's effects on the body's immune function can have far-reaching and lasting health consequences.

7.2.1 Incidence and Prevalence

Literature up until 2018 reported that there has been a general increase in the incidence of BP over the past two decades even before the pandemic, showing a 1.9- to 4.3-fold rise [9, 15]. The reason for this was attributed to various factors such as increasing life expectancy, more cases of neurological disorders that often occur alongside BP, growing use of medications known to trigger BP, particularly DPP4 inhibitors and psychiatric drugs and improved ability to diagnose the condition through better medical techniques.

The COVID-19 pandemic has since added another layer of complexity to this landscape [16, 17]. The full scope of post-COVID autoimmune manifestations remained unclear despite numerous case reports and small series. Two large-scale studies now highlight that SARS-CoV-2 infection is linked to a substantially increased risk of developing a diverse spectrum of new-onset autoimmune diseases. 19 conditions and in particular, new-onset autoimmune and inflammatory diseases in individuals who have had COVID-19 [18].

As for the role of COVID-19 infection in new onset BP, although there is evidence that SARS-

Cov-2 can stimulate autoantibody production inducing autoimmune diseases, existing literature reports very few cases of COVID -19- infection induced new onset AIBP.

7.2.2 Disease Exacerbation

Predisposing factors of BP development include genetics, comorbidities, and aging. Precipitating factors, such as drugs, vaccines, infections, physical factors and transplantation, refer to a specific event or trigger that could induce or exacerbate BP disease in the context of several predisposing factors [3].

Existing literature reports very few cases of COVID -19 induced flares and shows that it is improbable that COVID infection on its own worsens BP. Instead, most literature seems to focus on the risk of having severe forms of COVID-19 infection on BP patients and whether it affects the mortality rate in BP patients who have COVID-19-infection, which is discussed later in this chapter.

7.2.3 Diagnosis Challenges

The pandemic has led to challenges in diagnosing Bullous Pemphigoid due to the overlapping symptoms between COVID-19 and Bullous Pemphigoid. For instance, the appearance of blisters, which is a hallmark of Bullous Pemphigoid, can sometimes be confused with cutaneous manifestations of COVID-19 or its related conditions. The increased use of telemedicine during the pandemic also posed diagnostic challenges, as dermatologic assessments are often difficult to conduct remotely. Consequently, some patients with Bullous Pemphigoid may have faced delays in receiving appropriate care.

7.3 Effects of COVID-19 Vaccination on Bullous Pemphigoid

Recent literature present both new onset and reactivation of BP after SARS-CoV-2 vaccines [12, 19, 20]. A registry based study by McMohan et al [21] looked at 58 biopsy confirmed SARS-CoV-2-vaccine-associated cutaneous reactions of which BP-like lesions accounted for 20% (12/58). Another large multicentre study reported 21 cases of COVID19 vaccine associated BP and investigated this group's demographic, clinical and immunopathological patterns [22] . However, studies on exact pathways through which COVID-19 vaccines trigger Bullous Pemphigoid remain limited although several potential mechanisms, discussed in the next sections, have been proposed [4, 6, 22]. Despite these theories, more research is essential to definitively understand

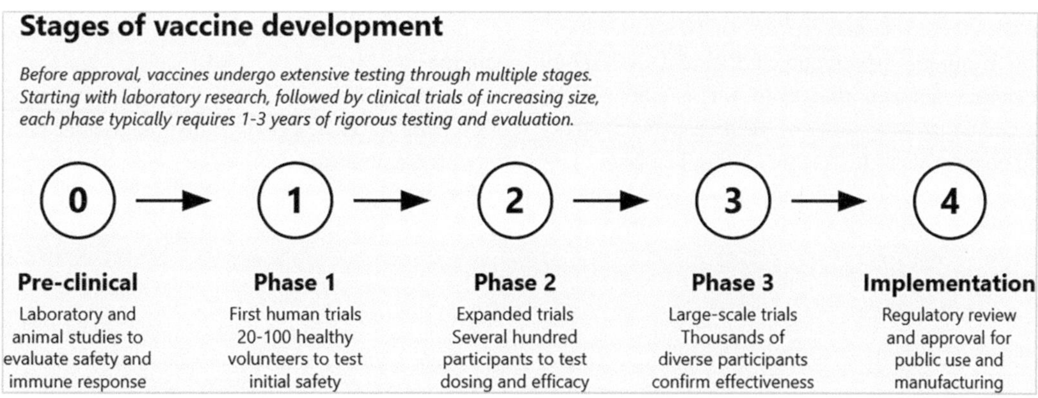

Fig. 7.6 Outlines the typical steps in vaccine development, from pre-clinical research to implementation, which can take several years to complete

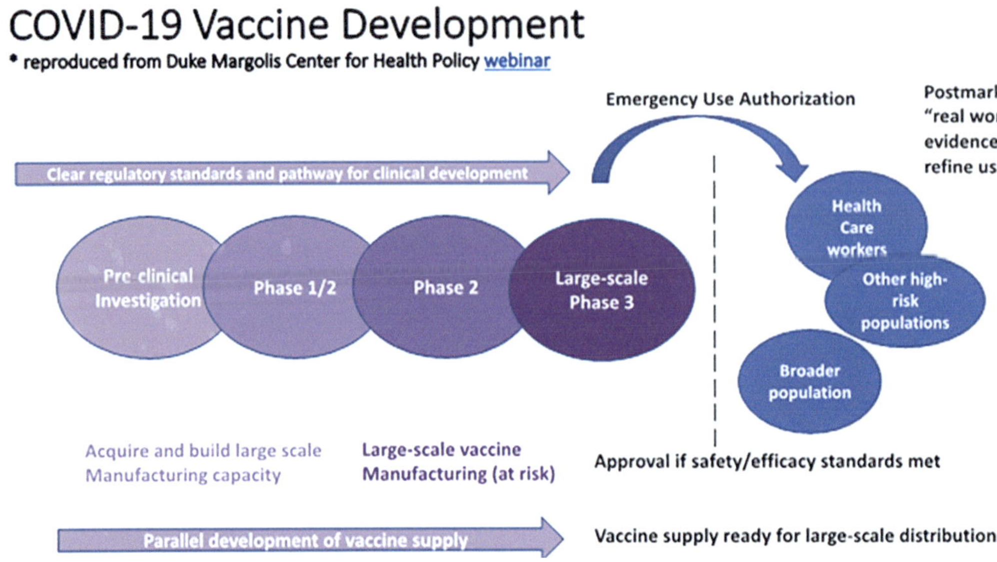

Fig. 7.7 COVID-19 vaccine development

how COVID-19 vaccines might trigger BP development.

7.3.1 Vaccine Safety and Bullous Pemphigoid

COVID-19 vaccines have been subject to rigorous safety evaluations (Fig. 7.6), and data suggest that they are generally safe for patients with autoimmune diseases [23], including Bullous Pemphigoid. However, as with any medical intervention, there have been isolated reports of autoimmune disease flare-ups following vaccination and a 2024 systematic review of 40 articles looking at patients who received different COVID-19 vaccines showed that even those who experienced a rare worsening of the disease were easily managed without further complications. This study also noted that onset on BP was more reported post-mRNA vaccines (especially the first dose of BNT162b2 vaccine, especially the first dose), particularly in the elderly population.

Notably, however there have been several reports of BP patients experiencing recurrences post vaccination during remission periods. However, the latency period from last dose of COVID-19 vaccination to BP flare was significantly varied and ranged from 3 to 45 days and so no causal link can be made.

Figure 7.7 focuses on the accelerated COVID-19 vaccine development, highlighting the emergency use authorization and the ramp-up of large-scale manufacturing to meet global demand.

These instances are still relatively rare and often need to be weighed against the overall benefits of vaccination.

7.3.2 COVID-19 Vaccine Types: Components and Clinical Considerations (Table 7.1)

7.3.3 Key Clinical Considerations

1. **Common Effects:** All vaccine types can cause temporary, mild-to-moderate effects such as injection site pain, fatigue, headache, muscle pain, and fever. These are generally signs of the immune system's response.
2. **Allergic Reactions:** PEG (in mRNA vaccines) and polysorbate 80 (in viral vector and some protein subunit vaccines) are most often linked to rare severe allergic reactions.
3. **Rare Specific Effects:**
   - mRNA vaccines: Myocarditis/pericarditis (more common in young males)
   - Adenovirus vector vaccines: Thrombosis with thrombocytopenia sy.ndrome (very rare)
4. **Autoimmune Considerations:**
   - Molecular Mimicry: Theoretical concern that similarity between viral and human proteins could trigger autoimmune responses, but no causal link established
   - Spike Protein: Present in all vaccine types, subject of ongoing research regarding potential autoimmune effects
   - Adjuvants: While crucial for vaccine efficacy, some debate exists about their long-term effects on the immune system
5. **Risk-Benefit Assessment:** For all authorised vaccines, the benefits of vaccination in preventing COVID-19 and its complications significantly outweigh known risks for most individuals.

Table 7.1 Highlights different types of vaccines against COVID-19, its components and potential safety considerations

Vaccine type	Examples	Key components	Potential effects and safety considerations
mRNA Vaccines	Pfizer-BioNTech, Moderna	mRNA encoding SARS-CoV-2 spike protein, Lipid nanoparticles, Polyethylene glycol (PEG), Salts, sugars	**PEG:** Rare cases of anaphylaxis **mRNA/Spike Protein**: Myocarditis/pericarditis (rare, typically mild, more common in young males) Theoretical concern for molecular mimicry (no causal link established) **Lipid Nanoparticles:** May contribute to reactogenicity (fever, chills, fatigue)
Viral vector vaccines	Oxford-AstraZeneca, Johnson & Johnson	Adenovirus vector, DNA encoding SARS-CoV-2 spike protein, Polysorbate 80, Salts, stabilizers	**Adenovirus Vector:** Rare thrombosis with thrombocytopenia syndrome (TTS) Rare cases of immune thrombocytopenia **Polysorbate 80**: Potential allergic reactions (less common than PEG) **Spike Protein**: Theoretical concern for molecular mimicry (no causal link established)
Protein subunit vaccines	Novavax	Recombinant SARS-CoV-2 spike protein, Matrix-M adjuvant (saponin-based), Polysorbate 80	**Adjuvant:** May increase local and systemic reactogenicity **Polysorbate 80**: Potential allergic reactions (rare), **Spike Protein**: Theoretical concern for molecular mimicry (no causal link established)
Inactivated virus vaccines	Sinovac, Bharat Biotech	Chemically inactivated SARS-CoV-2 virus, Aluminum-based adjuvants, Preservatives (e.g., thimerosal in multi-dose vials)	**Aluminium Adjuvants:** May increase local reactions (pain, swelling) Debated potential role in autoimmune phenomena **Preservatives:** Rare allergic reactions **Whole Virus Particles:** Theoretical potential for diverse immune responses

6. **Ongoing Surveillance:** Continuous safety monitoring helps identify and evaluate rare side effects and potential autoimmune phenomena that may emerge over time.
7. **Pre-existing Conditions:** Patients with autoimmune disorders or other pre-existing conditions should consult their healthcare providers for personalised advice, but generally, the benefits of vaccination outweigh potential risks.

7.3.4 Mechanisms Behind Vaccine-Triggered BP

Several theories attempt to explain what triggers bullous pemphigoid (BP) flare-ups, both in new cases and existing ones [4, 6, 22]. One hypothesis suggests that the SARS-CoV-2 spike protein might mimic certain proteins found in the skin's basement membrane, specifically BP-180 and BP-230 [6]. However, this seems unlikely since natural COVID-19 infections, which expose the body to the spike protein, haven't been shown to trigger BP.

Another theory focuses on how mRNA vaccines might affect people who are already prone to immune system problems. In these individuals, the vaccine's genetic material might activate specific immune receptors (TLRs 3, 7, and 8) [22], potentially triggering inflammation. This idea is supported by the discovery of COVID-19 vaccine-reactive T-cells in skin samples from a few BP patients who developed symptoms after vaccination.

These mechanisms might also explain why some patients taking certain medications (like blood pressure drugs, salicylates, and diuretics) develop BP after vaccination [3]- the vaccine might create conditions that make drug-induced BP more likely.

However, it's important to note that none of these explanations has been conclusively proven through rigorous scientific research.

7.3.5 Reported Cases of BP Post-COVID-19 Vaccination

New Onset BP

New-onset bullous pemphigoid may develop following COVID-19 vaccination [5, 6, 24, 25]. After ruling out other potential triggers for bullous pemphigoid, including drugs and other vaccinations, affected individuals should be monitored closely following subsequent COVID-19 vaccinations. Entering a period of clinical remission before pursuit of subsequent vaccinations should be considered to lessen the risk of a worsening cutaneous reaction.

Mortality

According to a Population-Based Study including 1845 BP patients, while BP patients do not appear to have an increased risk of contracting COVID-19 or requiring hospitalisation, they do face a higher risk of COVID-19-associated mortality, particularly in older age groups (>80 years old) [26].

7.3.6 Impact on Disease Management

BP is typically treated with corticosteroids and immunosuppressants, such as azathioprine and mycophenolate mofetil. This raised concerns because Autoimmune Bullous Disorders such as BP are generally vulnerable to opportunistic infections, especially infections like COVID19 pneumonia driving up mortality rates in BP patients. Especially old aged patients with comorbidities, may be at higher risk of poor outcomes of COVID-19 [27]. On the other hand, it has been postulated that immune system overactivation is responsible for the lung injury caused by SARS-CoV-2 and that a subgroup of patients might actually benefit from immunosuppressive drugs [14. This section discusses the challenges and considerations in treating BP during the pandemic.

7.3.7 Implications for Treatment

1. **Continuation of Therapy:**
   - Evidence supports maintaining BP-related therapies during the pandemic.
   - No significant association found between systemic corticosteroids or immunosuppressants and COVID-19 severity.

2. **Monitoring and Precautions:**
   - BP patients, especially those over 80, should be monitored closely if they develop COVID-19.
   - Enhanced precautions and adherence to safety measures are crucial for BP patients.
     - Enforce strict social distancing and discourage attendance at gatherings
     - Utilise teledermatology for remote consultations when possible
     - Regularly screen patients for COVID-19 symptoms
     - Assess patients' psychological well-being during periods of isolation, with special attention to those on high-dose corticosteroids
3. **Risk Stratification:**
   - Age appears to be a more significant factor than medication use in predicting COVID-19 outcomes for BP patients
   - Confirmed cases of COVID-19 should undergo risk evaluation at first and these drugs are only discontinued in proven cases of active COVID-19 after an individual risk-benefit analysis [17]
4. **Healthcare System Recommendations:**
   - Implement outreach programs to ensure the well-being of BP patients.
   - Hospitals should notify community healthcare personnel about the excess mortality risk in BP patients upon discharge.

7.3.8 Treatment Modifications

1. **Corticosteroids:**
   - Continue using the lowest effective dose.
   - Prednis(ol)one >10 mg/day may be reduced depending on the activity/severity of the AIBD, age, comorbidities and severity of COVID-19 in collaboration between the dermatologist and physician treating COVID-19.
   - No evidence to support discontinuation based on COVID-19 risk alone.
2. **Immunomodulators:**
   - Immunomodulating medications that are considered to impose the highest risks in patients with COVID-19 are azathioprine, mycophenolate mofetil/sodium, cyclophosphamide, and methotrexate [17]
   - May be stopped for the duration of COVID-19 symptoms, whereas topical corticosteroids, prednis(ol)one ≤10 mg/day, dapsone/sulphapyridine, doxycycline/tetracycline, colchicine and IVIG can be continued [17].
   - Individual risk-benefit analysis recommended for each patient.
3. **Topical Treatments:**
   - Emphasise the use of topical corticosteroids where possible.
   - Generally safer than systemic immunosuppression.
4. **Intravenous Immunoglobulin (IVIG):**
   - Remains a potential option for severe cases unresponsive to other treatments.
   - May have dual benefits in BP and COVID-19.
   - In BP patients with COVID-19 who are unresponsive to low-dose corticosteroids and/or antimicrobials and dapsone, this therapeutic option can be considered [17].
   - Potential side effects, particularly thromboembolism, should be considered [27].

7.4 Conclusion

The impact of COVID-19 and its vaccines on bullous pemphigoid (BP) management presents a complex medical scenario [16]. While the pandemic has brought challenges, including disease flare-ups and diagnostic hurdles, COVID-19 vaccines have generally proven beneficial for BP patients, with their protective benefits against severe COVID-19 outweighing potential risks. However, healthcare providers need to be aware that some individuals may develop new BP cases following COVID-19 vaccination.

A balanced approach to patient care is essential: carefully evaluating other possible BP triggers (including medications and other vaccines), while also recognizing the importance of COVID-19 protection [4, 6, 22]. For patients who develop BP after vaccination, careful monitoring during subsequent vaccine doses is crucial.

Ideally, these patients should achieve clinical remission before receiving additional COVID-19 vaccines to minimise the risk of skin reactions. This strategic approach, combined with ongoing research and vigilant monitoring, helps ensure optimal care for patients with autoimmune conditions in our evolving healthcare landscape.

References

1. Vaillant L, Bernard P, Joly P, Prost C, Labeille B, Bedane C, et al. Evaluation of clinical criteria for diagnosis of Bullous Pemphigoid. Arch Dermatol [Internet]. 1998 [cited 2020 Mar 5];134(9):1075–80. Available from: https://jamanetwork.com/journals/jamadermatology/fullarticle/189384
2. Bernard P, Antonicelli F. Bullous Pemphigoid: a review of its diagnosis, associations and treatment. Am J Clin Dermatol. 2017;18:513–28. https://doi.org/10.1007/s40257-017-0264-2.
3. Moro F, Fania L, Sinagra JLM, Salemme A, Zenzo GD. Bullous Pemphigoid: trigger and predisposing factors. Biomolecules [Internet]. 2020;10(10). Available from: https://pubmed.ncbi.nlm.nih.gov/33050407/
4. Cozzani E, Gasparini G, Russo R, Parodi A. May Bullous Pemphigoid be worsened by COVID-19 vaccine? Front Med [Internet]. 2022 [cited 2024 Nov 22];9. Available from: https://pmc.ncbi.nlm.nih.gov/articles/PMC9663456/
5. Aashish RA, Khatri G, Priya, Hasan MM. Bullous Pemphigoid following COVID-19 vaccine: an autoimmune disorder. Ann Med Surg. 2022;80:104266.
6. Wan V, Chen D, Shiau CJ, Jung GW. Association between COVID-19 vaccination and Bullous Pemphigoid—a case series and literature review. SAGE Open Medical Case Reports [Internet]. 2022 [cited 2024 Nov 22];10:2050313X2211318-8. Available from: https://ncbi.nlm.nih.gov/pmc/articles/PMC9580082/
7. Oakley A. Bullous Pemphigoid | DermNet NZ [Internet]. dermnetnz.org. 2016. Available from: https://dermnetnz.org/topics/bullous-pemphigoid
8. Mayo Clinic. Pemphigus—symptoms and causes [Internet]. Mayo Clinic. 2018. Available from: https://www.mayoclinic.org/diseases-conditions/pemphigus/symptoms-causes/syc-20350404
9. Kridin K, Ludwig RJ. The growing incidence of Bullous Pemphigoid: overview and potential explanations. Front Med. 2018;5.
10. Aref Ghanaatpisheh, Safari M, Hoda Haghshenas, Motamed-Sanaye A, Amir Homayoun Atefi, Karo Kamangarpour, et al. New-onset or flare-up of Bullous Pemphigoid associated with COVID-19 vaccines: a systematic review of case report and case series studies. Front Med [Internet]. 2024 [cited 2024 Dec 16];11. Available from: https://pmc.ncbi.nlm.nih.gov/articles/PMC11036870/
11. Olson N, Eckhardt D, Delano A. New-onset Bullous Pemphigoid in a COVID-19 patient. Case Rep Dermatol Med. 2021;2021:5575111. https://doi.org/10.1155/2021/5575111.
12. Rosińska-Wieckowicz A, Jałowska M, Bowszyc-Dmochowska M, Dmochowski M. Case report: infantile Bullous Pemphigoid: triggering by COVID 19 is speculative. Front Med. 2021;8:760823. https://doi.org/10.3389/fmed.2021.760823.
13. Pitlik SD. COVID-19 compared to other pandemic diseases. Rambam Maimonides Med J [Internet]. 2020;11(3):e0027. Available from: https://www.ncbi.nlm.nih.gov/pmc/articles/PMC7426550/
14. Winchester NE, Calabrese C, Calabrese L. The intersection of COVID-19 and autoimmunity: what is our current understanding? Pathogens Immunity. 2021;6(1):31–54.
15. Lu L, Chen L, Xu Y, Liu A. Global incidence and prevalence of Bullous Pemphigoid: a systematic review and meta-analysis. J Cosmetic Dermatol. 2022.
16. Drenovska K, Vassileva S, Tanev I, Joly P. Impact of COVID-19 on autoimmune blistering diseases. Clin Dermatol. 2021.
17. Azimi SZ, Firooz A, Murrell DF, Daneshpazhooh M. Treatment concerns for Bullous Pemphigoid in the COVID -19 pandemic era. Dermatol Ther. 2020.
18. Sharma C, Bayry J. High risk of autoimmune diseases after COVID-19. Nature Rev Rheumatol. 2023;19.
19. McMahon DE, Amerson E, Rosenbach M, Lipoff JB, Moustafa D, Tyagi A, Desai SR, French LE, Lim HW, Thiers BH, et al. Cutaneous reactions reported after Moderna and Pfizer COVID-19 vaccination: a registry-based study of 414 cases. J Am Acad Dermatol. 2021;85(1):46–55. https://doi.org/10.1016/j.jaad.2021.03.092.
20. Damiani G, Pacifico A, Pelloni F, Iorizzo M. The first dose of COVID-19 vaccine may trigger pemphigus and bullous pemphigoid flares: is the second dose therefore contraindicated? J Eur Acad Dermatol Venereol. 2021;35(10):e645. https://doi.org/10.1111/jdv.17472.
21. McMahon DE, Kovarik CL, Damsky W, et al. Clinical and pathologic correlation of cutaneous COVID-19 vaccine reactions including V-REPP: a registry-based study. J Am Acad Dermatol. 2022;86(1):113–21. https://doi.org/10.1016/j.jaad.2021.09.002.
22. Maronese CA, Caproni M, Moltrasio C, Genovese G, Vezzoli P, Sena P, Previtali G, Cozzani E, Gasparini G, Parodi A, Atzori L, Antiga E, Maglie R, Moro F, Mariotti EB, Corrà A, Pallotta S, Didona B, Marzano AV, Di Zenzo G. Bullous pemphigoid associated with COVID-19 vaccines: an italian multicentre study. Front Med. 2022;9:841506. https://doi.org/10.3389/fmed.2022.841506.

23. Tzioufas AG, Bakasis A-D, Goules AV, Bitzogli K, Cinoku II, Chatzis LG, Argyropoulou OD, Venetsanopoulou AI, Mavrommati M, Stergiou IE, Pezoulas V, Voulgari PV, Katsimpari C, Katechis S, Gazi S, Katsifis G, Sfontouris CI, Georgountzos AI, Liossis S-N, Papagoras C, Fotiadis DI, Skopouli FN, Vlachoyiannopoulos PG, Moutsopoulos HM. A prospective multicenter study assessing humoral immunogenicity and safety of the mRNA SARS-CoV-2 vaccines in Greek patients with systemic autoimmune and autoinflammatory rheumatic diseases. J Autoimmun. 2021;125:102743. https://doi.org/10.1016/j.jaut.2021.102743.
24. Olson N, Eckhardt D, Delano A. New-onset Bullous Pemphigoid in a COVID-19 patient. Case Rep Dermatol Med [Internet]. 2021;2021:1–6. Available from: https://pubmed.ncbi.nlm.nih.gov/34211788/
25. Pérez-López I, Moyano-Bueno D, Ruiz-Villaverde R. Bullous Pemphigoid and COVID-19 vaccine. Med Clín (English Edition). 2021;157(10):e333–4.
26. Kridin K, Schonmann Y, Weinstein O, Schmidt E, Ludwig RJ, Cohen AD. The risk of COVID-19 in patients with Bullous Pemphigoid and pemphigus: a population-based cohort study. J Am Acad Dermatol. 2021;85(1):79–87.
27. Chen J, Mao X, Zhao W, Zhang B, Chen X, Yu C, et al. Assessment of the characteristics and associated factors of infectious complications in Bullous Pemphigoid. Front Immunol. 2020;11.

8 The Effect of Covid-19 and Systemic Sclerosis

Karthi Kishore, Siva Chaitanya Senapathi, and Esraa M. AlEdani

8.1 Introduction

In the year 2020, the world was grappling with the issue of COVID-19 pandemic which caused significant economic, social, and medical burdens worldwide. Delays in clinical care, including new consultations, follow-up assessments, and treatment delivery, had posed significant concerns for patients globally. Among them were the patients being treated for rheumatic disorders. Systemic sclerosis (SSc), also known as scleroderma, is a chronic connective tissue disease characterized by fibrosis, vascular alterations, and autoantibody production. The onset of the COVID-19 pandemic had raised numerous questions regarding its interplay with Ssc among patients and healthcare providers owing to the complex nature of the disease. This chapter explores the impact of COVID-19 on patients with systemic sclerosis, including the risks, challenges, and management strategies.

8.2 Pathophysiology

The literature review states that there is are remarkable similarity between the pathogenesis of COVID 19 & SSc. The main triggers for COVID 19 infection were found to be viral exposure & subsequent infection. Similarly the triggers for SSc are environmental factors such as exposure to silica, vinyl chloride etc and genetic predisposition [1]. The fundamental pathogenic mechanism in SSc are vasculopathy, immune mechanism & fibrosis. It is prudent to know the relation of COVID 19 with each of this mechanism to establish its relationship with SSc.

(i) **VASCULOPATHY**

Though COVID 19 was initially identified as a respiratory illness, the presence of underlying vasculopathy was demonstrated at a later stage. The prevalence of thromboembolic disease in the form of pulmonary emboli and intravascular thrombosis was demonstrated in various stages of the disease, which may have contributed to the hypoxic symptoms of the disease. There is an underlying endothelial activation in the disease process responsible for clinical manifestation such as acrocyanosis and perniotic lesions of extremities ("Covid toes") which are akin to those seen in SSc [2]. The other mechanism of vasculopathy was the direct role of viral activation via ACE2 protein expressed on endothelial

K. Kishore (✉) · S. C. Senapathi
Department of Dermatology, Military Hospital, Shillong, Meghalaya, India

E. M. AlEdani
University of Basrah-Medical Faculty, Basrah, Iraq

E. M. AlEdani, H. Maibach (eds.), *COVID-19 Vaccination and Dermatological Diseases*, Updates in Clinical Dermatology, https://doi.org/10.1007/978-3-031-87791-9_8

cells causing subsequent coagulopathy and complement mediated damage [3]. The sequel of such changes can be demonstrated easily at the level of microcirculation using nailfold capillaroscopy showing reduced capillary density and haemorrhages which is a hallmark feature of early/active SSc [4].

(ii) **IMMUNE MECHANISM**

The disruption in the system of normal immune response and cytokine production is the main pathomechanism associated with development of immune mediated disease like SSc. The excessive immunological activation with failure to switch off signals that facilitate normal repair and regeneration is noticed in such conditions. There may be activation of pathways via innate immune system involving damage associated molecular patterns (DAMPs) or activation of interferon pathways or stimulation of adaptive immune system by viral antigens [5]. In context of COVID 19, the intrinsic factors of inflammation decides how effective the immune response to viral infection helps in elimination of virus and curtailing tissue damage. The same mechanism comes into play while deciding the clinical patterns & outcomes of SSc [5].

(iii) **FIBROSIS**

Systemic sclerosis is a pro- fibrotic disease whose pathogenic processes linked to vasculopathy and immuno-inflammation may lead to scarring of damaged organs. This may be especially relevant in the case of lungs where there is reduced capacity for tissue repair and regeneration that occurs in other organs. Based on clinical data, fibrosis is a recognised manifestation of COVID 19, where up to 25% of cases develop interstitial lung fibrosis and exhibit residual computed tomography (CT) abnormalities that persist even after the initial acute infection in COVID-19 [6]. The key mediator in SSc may be also seen in acute lung injury in COVID 19 which may include transforming growth factor (TGF-β), interleukin-6 (IL6), connective tissue growth factor (CTGF) and downstream pathways that lead to increased activation of myofibroblasts, excessive extracellular matrix (ECM) deposition or failure of appropriate ECM breakdown (Fig. 8.1).

Fig. 8.1 Successive endothelial cells alteration in COVID-19 and in systemic sclerosis (SSc). Although the pace of vascular changes is strikingly different (acute in COVID-19 and chronic in SSc), the two tracks share common pathologic alterations that trigger similar pathways and molecules with similar pathologic consequence. In the early stages, both pathways share functional EC changes including increase in vascular permeability, adhesion molecule expression, platelet activation, coagulation, microthrombosis, fibrinolysis and increased D-dimer and PAI-1 levels. Yet, each pathway has unique characteristics as noted in the prominence of vascular fibrotic changes and diminished angiogenesis in SSc and enhanced angiogenesis and macrothrombosis in COVID-19. The initial trigger in SSc is not known but viral, environmental (silica), and antibodies all can lead to functional and ultrastructural changes resulting in EC apoptosis, In COVID-19, direct EC invasion by SARS-CoV-2 and inflammasome activation triggering neutrophils adhesion, and the formation of neutrophil extracellular traps that damage endothelial further culminating in EC pyroptosis. It is assumed that autoimmune reaction and the generation of autoantibodies follows pyroptosis, while both are very prominent early in SSc. The resulting vascular disorder is more fibrotic in SSc and more thrombotic in COVID. Nonetheless, the impact on surrounding tissues is the same with prominent tissue ischemia and organ underperfusion. (Image courtesy: Marco Matucci-Cerinic, Michael Hughes, Gloria Taliani, Bashar Kahaleh, Similarities between COVID-19 and systemic sclerosis early vasculopathy: A "viral" challenge for future research in scleroderma, Autoimmunity Reviews, Volume 20, Issue 10, 2021)

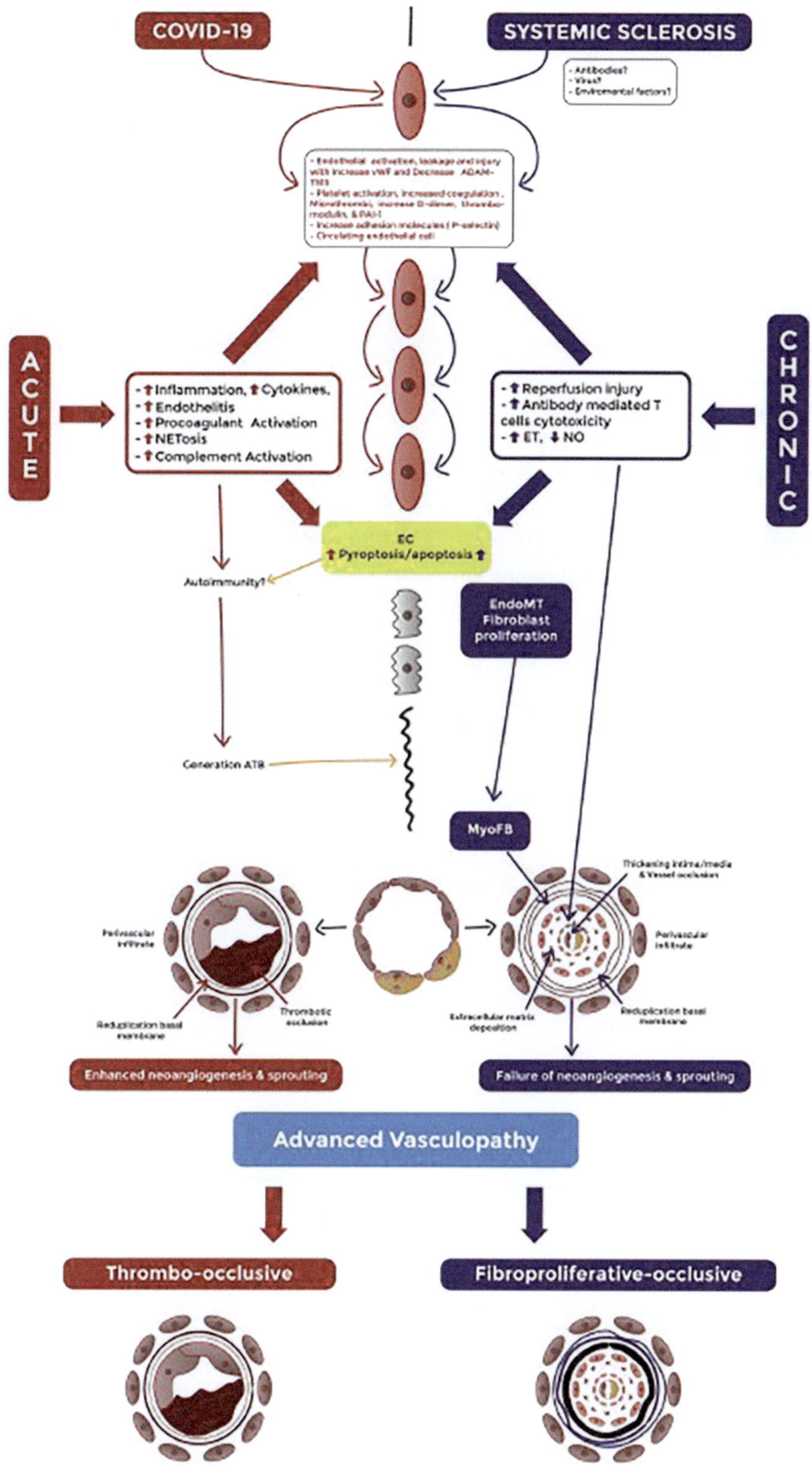
COVID-19
SYSTEMIC SCLEROSIS
- Antibodies?
- Virus?
- Environmental factors?
- Endothelial activation, leakage and injury with increase vWF and Decrease ADAM-TS13
- Platelet activation, increased coagulation,
- Increase adhesion molecules (P-selectin)
- Circulating endothelial cell
ACUTE
- ↑ Inflammation, ↑ Cytokines,
- ↑ Endothelitis
- ↑ Procoagulant Activation
- ↑ NETosis
- ↑ Complement Activation
CHRONIC
- ↑ Reperfusion injury
- ↑ Antibody mediated T cells cytotoxicity
- ↑ ET, ↓ NO
EC
↑ Pyroptosis/apoptosis ↑
Autoimmunity?
EndoMT
Fibroblast
proliferation
Generation ATB
MyoFB
Thickening intima/media & Vessel occlusion
Perivascular infiltrate
Reduplication basal membrane
Thrombotic occlusion
Extracellular matrix deposition
Perivascular infiltrate
Reduplication basal membrane
Enhanced neoangiogenesis & sprouting
Failure of neoangiogenesis & sprouting
Advanced Vasculopathy
Thrombo-occlusive
Fibroproliferative-occlusive

8.3 Clinical Features

The shared pathogenetic mechanisms of COVID-19 and SSc may pose risk to the patients in two ways :

(a) The negative impact of SSc on the course of COVID -19 & acceleration of underlying disease activity by the corona virus
(b) The emergence of new SSc manifestations [7]

8.4 Impact of COVID 19 on the Disease Activity in SSc & Vice Versa

The main symptoms of COVID 19 seen in patients of SSc was myalgia, arthralgia, fever, and cough. The patients with a pre existing interstitial lung disease(ILD) had a higher rate of diseases] activity & hospitalization (25.5%). It was noticed that patients with ILD & concomitant viral infection had a prolonged hospital stay and oxygen requirement. The various risk factors associated with poor outcome in concomitant COVID 19 infection are old age, male sex, non SSc comorbidities, associated ILD, renal or cardiac disease.

Guler et al stated that there was no evidence supporting the association between use of immunosuppressive agents such as rituximab, cyclophosphamide and corticosteroids with hospitalization and respiratory failure in COVID 19 [8]. The mortality from COVID 19 in SSc patients varied between 5% and 12% as per literature [9, 10]. There has been documented cases of emergence of SSc post COVID 19 infection and SARS-CoV-2 mRNA vaccination [11–14]. There has been increased incidence of Raynaud phenomenon and digital ulcers in patients of SSc post covid infection. There is a high risk of developing renal crisis in SSc due to administration of steroids for treating COVID. The SARS COV-2 infection causes acute lung injury along with inflammation and epithelial injury resulting in lung fibrosis and collagen deposition, which deteriorates lung disease in SSc [15–17]. There are case reports stating the emergence of de novo SSc & pre existing disease flare post SARS-CoV-2 infection (Table 8.1) [11–14].

Table 8.1 Key features showing the relationship between SSc and SARS-CoV-2 infection

The effect of COVID 19 on SSc	The effect of SSc on COVID 19
Increased disease activity	The increased requirement for oxygen and prolonged hospital stay
Onset of new disease/initial presentation post infection/ vaccination	Increased susceptibility to develop COVID infection in a pre existing SSc case
The aggravation of lung disease	Reduced sero-conversion and serum antibody concentration post COVID vaccination in people with pre existing disease
The increased incidence of Raynaud phenomenon and digital ulcers	
Increased incidence of Scleroderma renal crisis due to prolonged steroids	
Limited treatment options	

8.5 Management and Treatment Considerations for COVID-19 in Patients with Systemic Sclerosis

The management of COVID-19 in patients with systemic sclerosis (SSc) is quite challenging due to the autoimmune nature of SSc and the potential for severe disease manifestations. The various issues encountered while managing such cases are:

I. **CHALLENGES IN DIAGNOSIS AND MONITORING**

The patients with systemic sclerosis may present with overlapping symptoms of COVID-19 and their primary disease, such as dyspnoea, fatigue, and pulmonary involvement. The distinction between the two is essential for accurate diagnosis and timely intervention. High-resolution computed tomography (HRCT) scans and reverse transcription polymerase chain reaction (RT-PCR) tests for SARS-CoV-2 are essential diagnostic tools.

II. **THERAPEUTIC APPROACHES**

(i) **Immunosuppressive Therapy**

Systemic sclerosis patients are usually on long term immunosuppressives such as corticosteroids, methotrexate or biologics. In view of a concomitant COVID infection its imperative to ensure there is a balance between controlling SSc activity and minimizing infection risk. There might be a requirement for dose reduction or discontinuation of therapy while dealing with cases of severe COVID-19 infection [18].

(ii) **Antiviral and Anti-inflammatory Treatments**

The use of antiviral drugs like remdesivir and anti-inflammatory treatments such as dexamethasone has been shown to improve outcomes in COVID-19 patients. However, these treatments must be tailored to the individual needs of SSc patients, considering their underlying condition and concurrent medications [19].

(iii) **Respiratory Management**

Patients with systemic sclerosis are at increased risk of severe respiratory complications from COVID-19 due to pre-existing interstitial lung disease (ILD). Intensive monitoring of respiratory function and early intervention with supplemental oxygen, non-invasive ventilation, or mechanical ventilation may be required [10].

(iv) **Anticoagulation therapy**

SSc patients are at increased risk of thromboembolic events, a complication also observed in severe COVID-19. Prophylactic anticoagulation is recommended for hospitalized COVID-19 patients, and this practice should extend to those with SSc to mitigate the risk of thromboembolic complications [20].

III. **ADJUSTMENTS IN SYSTEMIC SCLEROSIS MANAGEMENT**

(i) **Monitoring and Follow-Up**

Frequent monitoring of SSc disease activity and COVID-19 symptoms is crucial. Telemedicine can be a valuable tool for regular follow-up while minimizing the risk of exposure to SARS-CoV-2 [21].

(ii) **Patient Education and Support**

Educating patients about the importance of adhering to preventive measures, recognizing early signs of COVID-19, and maintaining regular contact with healthcare providers is essential. It is noticed that patients of rheumatic disorders suffer from long term depression or anxiety, which seem to have been aggravated by the uncertainty imposed by the global pandemic. Providing psychological support to address anxiety and stress related to the pandemic and their chronic condition is also important [22].

IV. **VACCINATION ASPECTS**

Vaccination against COVID-19 is highly recommended for SSc patients, as it significantly reduces the risk of severe disease. Studies have shown that vaccines are generally safe and effective in this population, although there may be concerns regarding reduced immunogenicity due to concurrent immunosuppressive therapy. Adjustments in immunosuppressive regimens around the time of vaccination may be considered to enhance vaccine efficacy [23, 24].

8.6 Conclusion

Managing COVID-19 in patients with systemic sclerosis requires a multifaceted approach that considers the complexities of their autoimmune disease and the challenges posed by the pandemic. By adjusting immunosuppressive therapies, employing appropriate antiviral and anti-inflammatory treatments, and closely monitoring respiratory function, healthcare providers can improve outcomes for these vulnerable patients. Additionally, leveraging telemedicine and providing comprehensive patient education and support are critical components of effective management.

References

1. Figliozzi S, Masci PG, Ahmadi N, et al. Predictors of adverse prognosis in Covid-19: a systematic review andmeta-analysis. Eur J Clin Invest. 2020;29:e13362.
2. El Hachem M, Diociaiuti A, Concato C, et al. A clinical, histopathological and laboratory study of 19 consecutive Italian paediatric patients with chilblain-like lesions: lights and shadows on the relationship with COVID-19 infection. J Eur Acad Dermatol Venereol. 2020;34(11):2620–9.
3. Pons S, Fodil S, Azoulay E, et al. The vascular endothelium: the cornerstone of organ dysfunction in severe SARSCoV-2 infection. Crit Care. 2020;24:353.
4. Natalello G, De Luca G, Gigante L, et al. Nail fold capillaroscopy findings in patients with coronavirus disease 2019: broadening the spectrum of covid-19 microvascular involvement. Microvascular Research. 2020;133:104071.
5. Cardone M, Yano M, Rosenberg AS, et al. Lessons learned to date on COVID-19 hyperinflammatory syndrome: considerations for interventions to mitigate SARS-CoV-2 viral infection and detrimental hyperinflammation. Front Immunol. 2020;11:1131.
6. George PM, Wells AU, Jenkins RG. Pulmonary fibrosis and COVID-19: the potential role for antifibrotic therapy. Lancet Respir Med. 2020;8(8):807–15.
7. Denton CP, Campochiaro C, Bruni C, Distler O, Iagnocco A, et al. COVID-19 and systemic sclerosis: rising to the challenge of a pandemic. Journal of Scleroderma and Related Disorders. 2021;6(1):58–65.
8. Guler AA, Özçimen B, Aydoğdu MS, et al. Clinical characteristics and disease course before and after SARS-CoV-2 infection in a large cohort of systemic sclerosis patients. Turkish Journal of Medical Sciences. 2024;54(1):76–85. https://doi.org/10.55730/1300-0144.5768
9. de Oliveira SM, Martins LVO, Lupino-Assad AP, Medeiros- Ribeiro AC, de Moraes DA, et al. Severity and mortality of COVID-19 in patients with systemic sclerosis: a Brazilian multicenter study. Seminars in Arthritis and Rheumatism. 2022;55:151987. https://doi.org/10.1016/j.semarthrit.2022.151987.
10. Hoffmann-Vold AM, Brunborg C, Tirelli F, Carreira PE, Papa ND, et al. Impact and outcome of COVID-19 on SSc-ILD. European Respiratory Journal. 2021;58(suppl 65):PA2531. https://doi.org/10.1183/13993003.congress-2021.PA2531.
11. Fineschi S. Case report: systemic sclerosis after Covid-19 infection. Frontiers in Immunology. 2021;12:686699. https://doi.org/10.3389/fimmu.2021.686699.
12. Chandra A, Kahaleh B. Systemic Sclerosis (SSc) after COVID-19: a case report. Cureus. 2022;14(3):e23179. https://doi.org/10.7759/cureus.23179.
13. Campochiaro C, De Luca G, Farina N, Vignale D, Palmisano A, et al. Severe acute respiratory syndrome coronavirus-2- induced flare of systemic sclerosis. Scandinavian Journal of Rheumatology. 2022;51(2):156–8. https://doi.org/10.1080/03009742.2021.1932582.
14. Kondo M, Murakawa Y, Honda M, Moriyama M, Yoshioka Y A flare of systemic sclerosis potentially triggered by anti- SARS-CoV-2 mRNA vaccination. Rheumatol Adv Practice. 2022;6(3):rkac103. https://doi.org/10.1093/rap/rkac103.
15. Krygier A, Szmajda-Krygier D, Świechowski R, Pietrzak J, Wosiak A et al. Molecular pathogenesis of fibrosis, thrombosis and surfactant dysfunction in the lungs of severe COVID-19 patients. Biomolecules. 2022;12(12). https://doi.org/10.3390/biom12121845.
16. Zubieta-Calleja GR, Zubieta-DeUrioste N, de Jesús Montelongo F, Sanchez MGR, Campoverdi AF, et al. Morphological and functional findings in COVID-19 lung disease as compared to Pneumonia, ARDS, and High-Altitude Pulmonary Edema. Respiratory Physiology & Neurobiology. 2022;309:104000. https://doi.org/10.1016/j.resp.2022.104000.
17. Swarnakar R, Garje Y, Markandeywar N, Mehta S. Exploring the common pathophysiological links between IPF, SSc-ILD and post-COVID fibrosis. Lung India. 2022;39(3):279–85.
18. Furer V, Eviatar T, Zisman D, Peleg H, Paran D, Levartovsky D, et al. Immunosuppressive therapy and the risk of COVID-19 infection in patients with rheumatic diseases: a systematic review and meta-analysis. Semin Arthritis Rheum. 2020;50(5):927–34.

19. Beigel JH, Tomashek KM, Dodd LE, Mehta AK, Zingman BS, Kalil AC, et al. Remdesivir for the treatment of Covid-19—final report. N Engl J Med. 2020;383(19):1813–26.
20. Tang N, Bai H, Chen X, Gong J, Li D, Sun Z. Anticoagulant treatment is associated with decreased mortality in severe coronavirus disease 2019 patients with coagulopathy. J Thromb Haemost. 2020;18(5):1094–9.
21. Landewe RB, Machado PM, Kroon F, Bijlsma HWJ, Burmester GR, Carmona L, et al. EULAR provisional recommendations for the management of rheumatic and musculoskeletal diseases in the context of SARS-CoV-2. Ann Rheum Dis. 2020;79(7):851–8.
22. Hassen LM, Albarrak RA, Albahlal RA, et al. Functional and psychosocial impact of COVID-19 pandemic on rheumatic patients' quality of life in Saudi Arabia. Qual Life Res. 2022;31(11):3229–39. https://doi.org/10.1007/s11136-022-03184-1.
23. Geisen UM, Berner DK, Tran F, Sumbul M, Vullriede L, Ciripoi M, et al. Immunogenicity and safety of anti-SARS-CoV-2 mRNA vaccines in patients with chronic inflammatory conditions and immunosuppressive therapy in a monocentric cohort. Ann Rheum Dis. 2021;80(10):1306–11.
24. Buch MH, Eyre S, McGonagle D. Persistent antibody and T cell response to SARS-CoV-2 vaccination in patients with systemic autoimmune diseases on immunosuppression. Lancet Rheumatol. 2021;3(8).

9 The Effect of COVID-19 on Skin Cancer

Dimitra Xenopoulou and Esraa M. AlEdani

9.1 Overview

Individuals diagnosed with skin cancer face substantial risks, especially when undergoing treatments that compromise their immune systems. Essential therapies such as chemotherapy, immunotherapy, and radiation can significantly weaken the body's natural defenses, making patients more susceptible to infections, including COVID-19. This increased vulnerability underscores the urgent need for rigorous infection control measures and personalized healthcare management tailored specifically to protect these high-risk individuals. Effective infection prevention strategies and tailored treatment protocols are crucial to mitigating the compounded risks faced by these patients.

The COVID-19 pandemic has introduced a range of secondary risks due to public health measures, such as lockdowns and social distancing protocols. While these measures were critical for curbing the spread of the virus, they inadvertently disrupted routine dermatologic care, particularly skin cancer screenings. Many patients experienced delays, postponements, or cancellations of their dermatology appointments. These interruptions have had a profound impact, potentially leading to delays in the detection of new skin cancer cases and the monitoring of existing conditions. The ramifications of these delays are significant, as they may allow skin cancers to progress unchecked, resulting in more advanced disease stages by the time of eventual diagnosis. This progression could lead to more complex and challenging treatment scenarios, potentially impacting patient outcomes [1].

The temporary suspension or reduction of skin cancer screening programs during the pandemic, as healthcare resources were reallocated to address the immediate demands of COVID-19, has likely contributed to a decrease in the detection rate of new skin cancer cases. This decline in screening affects not only the prevalence of detected cases but also complicates the epidemiological understanding of skin cancer trends during the pandemic. With fewer screenings, delayed diagnoses and treatments may result in poorer outcomes, potentially increasing the long-term burden of skin cancer on both individual patients and the healthcare system [2].

In addition to these challenges, the pandemic has led to significant changes in lifestyle and behavior that have impacted sun exposure patterns. For some individuals, lockdowns and stay-at-home orders led to reduced outdoor activities, which may have decreased their risk of sun exposure. On the other hand, others increased their time outdoors as a means of recreation or exer-

D. Xenopoulou (✉)
New York Institute of Technology College of Osteopathic Medicine (NYITCOM), Old Westbury, NY, USA

E. M. AlEdani
University of Basrah-Medical Faculty, Basrah, Iraq

E. M. AlEdani, H. Maibach (eds.), *COVID-19 Vaccination and Dermatological Diseases*, Updates in Clinical Dermatology, https://doi.org/10.1007/978-3-031-87791-9_9

cise, potentially elevating their risk of skin cancer. These behavioral shifts have introduced complexity in understanding how the pandemic has influenced skin cancer incidence. The varied effects across different demographic groups highlight the need for ongoing research to determine the pandemic's overall impact on skin cancer trends [3].

Finally, the psychological toll of the pandemic, characterized by heightened stress and anxiety, cannot be overlooked. These mental health challenges may exacerbate pre-existing conditions, including skin cancer, and negatively influence treatment adherence and outcomes. Increased stress can affect patients' overall well-being and their ability to manage their health conditions effectively. Addressing these psychological aspects is essential in developing comprehensive healthcare strategies that prioritize not only the immediate health needs of patients but also their long-term well-being as they navigate the dual challenges of skin cancer and the COVID-19 pandemic. Ensuring support for mental health and well-being is crucial in providing holistic care and improving patient outcomes during these challenging times.

9.2 Innovative Strategies in Dermatologic Care: Managing Skin Cancer During the COVID-19 Pandemic

As healthcare systems worldwide grapple with the challenges posed by the COVID-19 pandemic, dermatologists and oncologists have played a crucial role in developing innovative strategies to ensure that care for skin cancer patients remains uninterrupted. One of the most significant advancements in this context is the widespread adoption of telemedicine. This approach has become essential during the pandemic, enabling virtual consultations, remote monitoring of treatment progress, and ongoing patient support without the need for in-person visits. By minimizing the risk of COVID-19 exposure for both patients and healthcare providers, telemedicine ensures that patients continue to receive critical medical guidance and intervention [4].

The integration of teledermatology has further enhanced patient care. Through the use of teledermoscopy, dermatologists can remotely examine suspicious skin lesions, assessing potential skin cancers from a distance. This technology leverages high-resolution images and real-time communication, allowing healthcare providers to identify and prioritize high-risk cases for in-person evaluations. As a result, urgent cases receive timely attention despite the restrictions imposed by the pandemic [5, 6].

In addition to technological innovations, it is essential for skin cancer patients to adhere strictly to preventive measures recommended by public health authorities. Patients undergoing treatments that suppress immune function are particularly vulnerable and must take proactive steps to prevent infection. Measures such as frequent handwashing, consistent mask usage in public spaces, and maintaining physical distance are vital for reducing the risk of contracting COVID-19. These precautions not only protect patients from the virus but also ensure that their cancer treatments proceed without unnecessary interruptions.

As healthcare systems adapt to the evolving challenges of the pandemic, efforts are also being made to restore and optimize dermatologic services for skin cancer patients. Strategies include prioritizing essential in-person consultations for high-risk individuals while managing less urgent cases remotely. This triage system helps ensure that patients receive timely care based on the severity of their condition, thereby reducing delays in diagnosis and treatment that could lead to worse outcomes [7, 8].

Healthcare providers are also engaging in public awareness campaigns to encourage individuals to seek medical attention for any concerning skin changes or symptoms, even during the pandemic. Empowering patients with knowledge about early signs and symptoms of skin cancer is crucial for facilitating early detection and intervention, which are key factors in improving survival rates and quality of life [9].

To further ensure patient safety, enhanced infection control protocols have been implemented within clinical settings. These include strict hygiene practices, regular sanitization of facilities, and optimized scheduling to minimize patient density and ensure adequate physical distancing during in-person visits. Such measures create a safe environment for both patients and healthcare staff, enabling the continuation of essential dermatologic care.

Navigating the intersection of skin cancer and the COVID-19 pandemic requires a concerted effort from healthcare providers, patients, and public health systems. By embracing telemedicine, adhering to preventive measures, and implementing rigorous infection control practices, the medical community can effectively manage skin cancer amidst the ongoing challenges posed by the pandemic, ensuring that patient care remains a top priority.

9.3 Impact of COVID-19 on Skin Cancer: Etiology, Pathophysiology, and Diagnosis

COVID-19 has profoundly influenced various aspects of skin cancer, including its etiology, pathophysiology, incidence, and prevalence. Understanding these impacts is crucial for managing skin cancer effectively during the ongoing pandemic.

9.3.1 Etiology

The COVID-19 pandemic has altered environmental and behavioral factors affecting skin cancer risk. Lockdowns and social distancing measures have led to significant changes in daily routines, impacting sun exposure patterns. Many people experienced reduced sun exposure due to increased indoor time, which might lower the risk of skin cancer associated with excessive sun exposure. However, this reduction was not uniform. For example, healthcare workers and essential personnel who continued working outside may have faced increased sun exposure during the pandemic. These contrasting experiences underscore the complexity of environmental influences on skin cancer risk during periods of societal disruption [10].

Additionally, the pandemic has influenced other behavioral factors related to skin cancer risk. Stress and lifestyle changes associated with COVID-19 may have altered patterns of self-care and health-seeking behaviors. Reduced access to dermatologic care during the pandemic has led to delays in routine skin checks and screenings, potentially resulting in missed or late diagnoses of skin cancer. These missed opportunities for early detection can have serious consequences for patient outcomes.

9.3.2 Immune Suppression

COVID-19, particularly in severe cases, is associated with significant immune dysregulation and suppression. Severe forms of the disease can induce a cytokine storm—a condition where the immune system releases an excessive amount of cytokines, leading to widespread inflammation. This overactive immune response is detrimental not only to respiratory health but also to overall immune function [11].

In the context of skin cancer, immune suppression due to severe COVID-19 presents several risks and challenges. The immune system plays a crucial role in recognizing and eliminating cancerous cells, including those involved in melanoma, basal cell carcinoma (BCC), and squamous cell carcinoma (SCC). Immune suppression can impair this surveillance and defense mechanism, allowing cancer cells to evade detection and proliferate. This impairment could potentially increase the likelihood of skin cancer development or exacerbate existing malignancies. Patients with predisposing factors for skin cancer—such as chronic sun exposure, use of immunosuppressive medications, or a history of skin cancer—are particularly vulnerable to the effects of COVID-19-induced immune suppression. Prolonged periods of immune compromise following severe COVID-19 could enhance skin cancer risk or worsen the prognosis of existing tumors. Additionally, chronic inflammation from a cytokine storm may create a pro-tumorigenic microenvironment within skin tumors, promoting cancer cell growth, angiogenesis (formation of new blood vessels), and metastasis. This inflammatory milieu underscores the need for comprehensive management strategies, including close monitoring of immune status and personalized risk assessment [12].

9.3.3 Pathophysiology

The pathophysiological impact of COVID-19 extends beyond respiratory manifestations, affecting immune regulation and inflammation—critical factors in skin cancer progression. The systemic inflammatory responses and immune dysregulation caused by COVID-19 can alter immune surveillance against skin cancer cells and the inflammatory microenvironment within tumors. These immunological shifts highlight the need for ongoing research to understand how COVID-19 may modulate the pathways involved in skin cancer. The pandemic has disrupted healthcare systems globally, leading to significant challenges in the timely diagnosis and treatment of various medical conditions, including skin cancer. Public health measures such as lockdowns, social distancing, and reallocation of healthcare resources have reduced access to dermatologic services and postponed screenings [13].

9.3.4 Delayed Diagnosis

One major consequence of the disrupted healthcare system during the pandemic has been delays in skin cancer detection. Routine dermatologic appointments, including screenings for suspicious lesions and follow-up visits for high-risk individuals, were often postponed or canceled to prioritize urgent COVID-19 care. These delays have resulted in prolonged intervals between recognizing symptoms and receiving definitive diagnostic evaluation.

Delayed diagnosis is particularly concerning for skin cancers, which can progress rapidly if left untreated. Early detection is crucial for melanoma, BCC, and SCC, as it allows for timely intervention and potentially curative treatments. The postponement of screenings may lead to a higher proportion of diagnoses at advanced stages, characterized by larger tumor sizes, deeper invasion into surrounding tissues, and increased likelihood of metastasis. This shift could impact overall survival rates and quality of life for skin cancer patients, making the need for timely diagnosis and treatment more critical than ever [14, 15].

9.3.5 Research and Collaboration

The scientific community is actively researching the relationship between COVID-19 and skin cancer. Preliminary studies suggest that individuals with skin cancer do not inherently face a higher risk of contracting COVID-19 compared to the general population. However, ongoing research is essential to fully understand how these two health challenges intersect and their impact on patient outcomes.

Researchers are exploring how COVID-19 may influence skin cancer prognosis and management. The virus's effects on immune function and systemic inflammation pose significant considerations for patients undergoing treatment. For instance, COVID-19's impact on immune responses might alter treatment efficacy or disease progression. Understanding these effects is crucial for developing tailored approaches that optimize both COVID-19 management and skin cancer care [16].

Additionally, researchers are investigating the broader implications of COVID-19 on individuals with pre-existing skin conditions like psoriasis and eczema. These conditions share immune dysregulation features with skin cancer and could influence the development or progression of malignancies. Insights into these interactions are vital for guiding comprehensive healthcare strategies during the pandemic.

As research continues, collaboration between dermatologists, oncologists, and infectious disease specialists becomes increasingly vital. By pooling expertise and data, the scientific community can accelerate discovery and develop more informed guidelines and treatment protocols, enhancing patient care and resilience amidst the complex interplay between COVID-19 and skin cancer [17].

9.4 Navigating Uncertainty and Building Resilience

The COVID-19 pandemic has presented unprecedented challenges for individuals managing skin cancer, necessitating a proactive and resilient approach. Effectively navigating this intersection requires open communication with healthcare providers, adherence to preventive measures, and the development of robust support systems to maintain both physical and emotional well-being.

9.4.1 Communication with Healthcare Providers

Maintaining open and consistent dialogue with healthcare providers is essential for individuals with skin cancer. Regular consultations allow for adjustments to treatment plans based on concerns related to COVID-19 and its impact on skin cancer management. This communication helps ensure continuity of care, facilitates timely modifications to treatment protocols, and provides reassurance during uncertain times. Addressing concerns about how COVID-19 might affect skin cancer care is vital for implementing strategies that prioritize patient safety while delivering effective treatment [18].

9.4.2 Preventive Measures

Adhering to preventive measures is crucial for minimizing the risk of COVID-19 transmission among individuals with skin cancer. Fundamental practices include rigorous hand hygiene, consistent mask-wearing in public spaces, and physical distancing. Additionally, self-monitoring for COVID-19 symptoms—such as fever, cough, or difficulty breathing—is essential. Prompt medical attention for any new or worsening symptoms ensures timely intervention, reducing the impact of COVID-19 on skin cancer care [19, 20].

9.4.3 Impact on Diagnosis and Treatment

The pandemic has significantly affected skin cancer incidence and prevalence through various mechanisms. Healthcare service disruptions, including delays in dermatologic screenings and elective procedures, have led to postponed or canceled appointments. These delays may result in missed opportunities for early detection, potentially increasing the number of advanced-stage diagnoses as the pandemic subsides. Conversely, heightened public awareness of health risks during the pandemic might have encouraged some individuals to seek dermatologic evaluations for concerning skin lesions, potentially influencing incidence trends [21].

9.4.4 Disruption of Treatment Pathways

The pandemic has also disrupted treatment pathways for those already diagnosed with skin cancer. Elective procedures, such as surgical excisions, Mohs surgery for basal cell carcinoma (BCC) and squamous cell carcinoma (SCC), and reconstructive surgeries, were frequently deferred to conserve healthcare resources and reduce COVID-19 transmission risks. This has led to extended waiting times for definitive treatments, which could impact disease progression and overall prognosis. Prolonged interruptions in treatment schedules might affect outcomes for those undergoing systemic therapies or radiation for advanced skin cancers. Ensuring continuity in treatment is crucial for achieving optimal outcomes and preventing recurrence or progression [22, 23].

9.4.5 Socioeconomic Impacts and Health Disparities

The socioeconomic impact of the pandemic has disproportionately affected vulnerable populations, exacerbating existing health disparities. Access to dermatologic care has been variably compromised, highlighting the need for equitable healthcare delivery strategies to address these disparities. Ensuring that all individuals, particularly those from disadvantaged backgrounds, have access to essential skin cancer services is crucial in mitigating the broader impacts of the pandemic on skin cancer outcomes [24].

9.4.6 Support and Self-Care

Building a robust support network is invaluable during these challenging times. Connecting with family, friends, or support groups provides emotional reinforcement and practical assistance. Seeking reliable information from trusted sources, such as healthcare professionals and reputable health organizations, helps individuals make informed decisions about their health amidst evolving circumstances. Prioritizing self-care is also vital. Maintaining a healthy lifestyle through balanced nutrition, regular exercise, and adequate rest supports physical health and resilience. Mindfulness practices, such as meditation and relaxation techniques, can help manage stress and anxiety, which may be heightened during the pandemic.

9.4.7 Adapting to Evolving Healthcare Landscapes

As individuals adapt to the changing healthcare landscape and infection control measures, resilience becomes a cornerstone of managing uncertainty. Embracing flexibility in treatment plans, leveraging telemedicine for virtual consultations, and staying informed about updates in medical guidelines are proactive steps to effectively manage the intersection of skin cancer and COVID-19. These strategies ensure continued access to essential care while mitigating risks [25, 26].

9.5 Conclusion

The convergence of COVID-19 and skin cancer highlights the profound interconnectedness of global health crises and underscores the need for a comprehensive approach to healthcare delivery. As we continue to navigate the challenges posed by the pandemic, prioritizing the needs of individuals with skin cancer remains crucial [27].

Addressing these intertwined health challenges demands a multifaceted strategy that embraces collaboration, innovation, and resilience. Healthcare professionals across various disciplines must work together to optimize care pathways for patients managing both COVID-19 and skin cancer. This collaborative approach not only enhances patient outcomes but also fosters a unified healthcare response that can adapt to evolving circumstances.

Innovation plays a key role in adapting to the changing landscape of healthcare during the pandemic. Technologies such as telemedicine have become indispensable, allowing for safe and effective remote consultations and monitoring. By embracing these advancements, healthcare providers can maintain continuity of care while minimizing exposure risks for vulnerable patients.

Resilience is essential for navigating the uncertainties brought about by these combined health crises. Empowering individuals with knowledge, providing steadfast support through dedicated healthcare teams, and promoting proactive health management strategies are crucial in mitigating the impact of both COVID-19 and skin cancer.

Looking ahead, our collective commitment to addressing these challenges will pave the way for a healthier future. Through ongoing research, education, and community engagement, we can strengthen healthcare systems and enhance preparedness for future health emergencies. Together, we can build a more resilient healthcare infrastructure that prioritizes comprehensive care and equitable access for all individuals affected by skin cancer and other complex health conditions [28].

As we move forward, let us remain steadfast in our dedication to improving health outcomes, fostering innovation, and promoting global health equity. By uniting in our pursuit of excellence in healthcare, we can navigate these unprecedented times with compassion, determination, and hope.

In summary, the COVID-19 pandemic has reshaped the landscape of skin cancer management by impacting diagnostic and treatment pathways, exacerbating health disparities, and emphasizing the importance of resilience and self-care. Addressing these evolving dynamics requires ongoing research, vigilant surveillance, and targeted interventions to optimize skin cancer prevention, detection, and management in the post-pandemic era. By maintaining open communication with healthcare providers, adhering to preventive measures, and fostering supportive networks, individuals can navigate the challenges of managing skin cancer during the pandemic with greater confidence and resilience [29].

COVID-19 has introduced new challenges and complexities in the realm of skin cancer, affecting its etiology, pathophysiology, incidence, and prevalence. Proactive measures are essential to ensure timely diagnosis, treatment, and support for individuals affected by skin cancer throughout the ongoing pandemic and beyond [30].

References

1. Aryanian Z, Balighi K, Goodarzi A, Sadeghi Nia A, Afshar ZM, Hatami P. The impact of the COVID-19 pandemic on the diagnosis and treatment of skin cancers, a mini review. Cancer Rep (Hoboken). 2023;6(9). https://doi.org/10.1002/cnr2.1854.
2. Tejera-Vaquerizo A, Paradela S, Toll A, et al. Effects of COVID-19 lockdown on tumour burden of melanoma and cutaneous squamous cell carcinoma. Acta Derm Venereol. 2021;101(8). https://doi.org/10.2340/00015555-3890.
3. Sacchetto L, Zanetti R, Comber H, Bouchardy C, Brewster DH, Broganelli P, et al. Trends in incidence of thick, thin and in situ melanoma in Europe. Eur J Cancer. 2018;92:108–18.
4. Carr BG, Hollander JE. Virtually perfect? Telemedicine for Covid-19. N Engl J Med. 2020;382(18):1679–81. https://doi.org/10.1056/NEJMp2003539.
5. Ibrahim AE, Magdy M, Khalaf EM, Mostafa A, Arafa A. Teledermatology in the time of COVID-19. Int J Clin Pract. 2021;75(12). https://doi.org/10.1111/ijcp.15000.
6. Jobbágy A, Kiss N, Meznerics FA, et al. Emergency use and efficacy of an asynchronous teledermatology system as a novel tool for early diagnosis of skin cancer during the first wave of COVID-19 pandemic. Int J Environ Res Public Health. 2022;19(5):2699. https://doi.org/10.3390/ijerph19052699.
7. Mashoudy KD, Perez SM, Nouri K. From diagnosis to intervention: a review of telemedicine's role in skin cancer care. Arch Dermatol Res. 2024;316(5):139. https://doi.org/10.1007/s00403-024-02884-7.
8. Tagliaferri L, Di Stefani A, Schinzari G, et al. Skin cancer triage and management during COVID-19 pandemic. J Eur Acad Dermatol Venereol. 2020;34(6):1136–9. https://doi.org/10.1111/jdv.16529.
9. Darlenski R, Tsankov N. COVID-19 pandemic and the skin: what should dermatologists know? Clin Dermatol. 2020;38(2):188.
10. Aguilera J, de Gálvez MV, Aguilera P, de Troya-Martín M, Gilaberte Y, del Grupo Español de Fotobiología de la AEDV. Recommendations on sun exposure and photoprotection following easing of the COVID-19 pandemic lockdown: Spanish Photobiology Group of the Spanish Academy of Dermatology and Venerology (AEDV). Actas Dermosifiliogr. 2020;111(9):799–801. https://doi.org/10.1016/j.adengl.2020.06.004.
11. Davitt E, Davitt C, Mazer MB, Areti SS, Hotchkiss RS, Remy KE. COVID-19 disease and immune dysregulation. Best Pract Res Clin Haematol. 2022;35(3):101401. https://doi.org/10.1016/j.beha.2022.101401.
12. Khayyati Kohnehshahri M, Sarkesh A, Mohamed Khosroshahi L, et al. Current status of skin cancers with a focus on immunology and immunotherapy. Cancer Cell Int. 2023;23(1):174. https://doi.org/10.1186/s12935-023-03012-7.
13. Brandão MGSA, Barros LM, de Aquino Mendonça J, de Oliveira AR, de Araújo TM, Veras VS. Clinical and histopathological findings of cutaneous manifestations of COVID-19 patients. Dermatol Ther. 2020;33(6). https://doi.org/10.1111/dth.13926.
14. Dessinioti C, Garbe C, Stratigos AJ. The impact of the COVID-19 pandemic on diagnostic delay of skin cancer: a call to restart screening activities. J Eur Acad Dermatol Venereol. 2021;35(12). https://doi.org/10.1111/jdv.17552.
15. Rashid S, Tsao H. Effect of the COVID-19 pandemic on delayed skin cancer services. Dermatol Clin. 2021;39(4):627–37. https://doi.org/10.1016/j.det.2021.05.015.
16. Cariti C, Merli M, Avallone G, et al. Melanoma management during the COVID-19 pandemic emergency: a literature review and single-center experience. Cancers (Basel). 2021;13(23):6071. https://doi.org/10.3390/cancers13236071.
17. Mostafavi Zadeh SM, Rezaei Y, Barahimi A, Abbasi E, Malekzadeh R. Impact of COVID-19 pandemic on the diagnosis of patients with skin cancer: a systematic review protocol. BMJ Open. 2023;13(3). https://doi.org/10.1136/bmjopen-2022-069720.
18. Drenovska K, Schmidt E, Vassileva S. Covid-19 pandemic and the skin. Int J Dermatol.

2020;59(11):1312–9. https://doi.org/10.1111/ijd.15189.
19. Jeremić J, Suđecki B, Radenović K, et al. Impact of the COVID-19 pandemic on melanoma diagnosis: increased breslow thickness in primary melanomas-a single center experience. Int J Environ Res Public Health. 2022;19(24):16806. https://doi.org/10.3390/ijerph192416806.
20. Rundle CW, Presley CL, Militello M, et al. Hand hygiene during COVID-19: recommendations from the American Contact Dermatitis Society. J Am Acad Dermatol. 2020;83(6):1730–7. https://doi.org/10.1016/j.jaad.2020.07.057.
21. Baumann BC, MacArthur KM, Brewer JD, et al. Management of primary skin cancer during a pandemic: multidisciplinary recommendations. Cancer. 2020;126(17):3900–6. https://doi.org/10.1002/cncr.32969.
22. Bhargava S, McKeever C, Kroumpouzos G. Impact of COVID-19 pandemic on dermatology practices: results of a web-based, global survey. Int J Womens Dermatol. 2021;7(2):217–23. https://doi.org/10.1016/j.ijwd.2020.09.010.
23. Tejera-Vaquerizo A, Cañueto J, Toll A, et al. Estimated effect of COVID-19 lockdown on skin tumor size and survival: an exponential growth model. Actas Dermosifiliogr (Engl Ed). 2020;111(8):629–38. https://doi.org/10.1016/j.ad.2020.05.001.
24. Andraska EA, Alabi O, Dorsey C, et al. Health care disparities during the COVID-19 pandemic. Semin Vasc Surg. 2021;34(3):82–8. https://doi.org/10.1053/j.semvascsurg.2021.08.002.
25. Brochez L, Baurain JF, Del Marmol V, et al. Recommendations for skin cancer consultation and surgery during COVID-19 pandemic. J Eur Acad Dermatol Venereol. 2020;34(9):1876–8. https://doi.org/10.1111/jdv.16772.
26. Desai SR, McMichael AJ, Khanna R. Coronavirus disease 2019 and race in dermatology. Dermatol Clin. 2021;39(4):569–74. https://doi.org/10.1016/j.det.2021.05.003.
27. Prasad S, Bassett IV, Freeman EE. Dermatology on the global stage: the role of dermatologists in international health advocacy and COVID-19 research. Int J Womens Dermatol. 2021;7(5):653–9. https://doi.org/10.1016/j.ijwd.2021.10.003.
28. Stoff BK, Blalock TW, Swerlick RA, MacKelfresh JB, Lawley LP, Chen SC. Guiding principles for prioritization of limited in-person dermatology appointments during the COVID-19 pandemic. J Am Acad Dermatol. 2020;83(4):1228–30. https://doi.org/10.1016/j.jaad.2020.07.024.
29. Geskin LJ, Trager MH, Aasi SZ, et al. Perspectives on the recommendations for skin cancer management during the COVID-19 pandemic. J Am Acad Dermatol. 2020;83(1):295–6. https://doi.org/10.1016/j.jaad.2020.05.002.
30. Venables ZC, Ahmed S, Bleiker OT, et al. The impact of the COVID-19 pandemic on skin cancer incidence and treatment in England, 2020. Br J Dermatol. 2021;185(2):460–2. https://doi.org/10.1111/bjd.20409.

The Effect of COVID-19 on Sézary Syndrome

10

Esraa M. AlEdani

10.1 Introduction

Sézary syndrome (SS) is a rare and aggressive form of cutaneous T-cell lymphoma (CTCL), characterized by the malignant presence of T-cells in the blood, skin, and lymph nodes. Patients with SS suffer from chronic, erythrodermic skin inflammation, pruritus, and immunodeficiency. Because the immune system is compromised, COVID-19 presents unique challenges for these individuals. The pandemic has not only increased the risk of severe outcomes for SS patients but also disrupted their ongoing medical care. This paper explores the intersection of COVID-19 and Sézary syndrome, focusing on the clinical outcomes, challenges in treatment, and potential future directions.

10.2 Overview of Sézary Syndrome (SS)

CTCL has a leukemic form known as Sezary syndrome. It manifests as symptoms like these:

Erythroderma: Skin that is red all over and scaly.

Pruritus: Excessive itching that compromises one's quality of life.

Enlarg lymph nodes: are known as lymphadenopathy.

Sezary cells: Unusual T-cells found in the bloodstream.

Systemic immunosuppression in SS patients makes them susceptible to infections. Therapies include phototherapy, immunosuppressants, chemotherapy, and biologic medicines can further suppress immune function while also trying to regulate symptoms and limit the progression of the disease [1].

10.3 Immunocompromised State and COVID-19 Risk in SS Patients

It is well recognized that COVID-19 disproportionately affects those with compromised immune systems, such as those suffering from cancer or long-term illnesses. Individuals who have Sézary syndrome are considered high-risk due to various factors:

Immune dysfunction: The cancerous T-cells interfere with the body's natural defenses, making it more difficult to fight off infections, such as SARS-CoV-2.

Immunosuppressive therapies: Treatments for sickle cell disease (SS), such as methotrexate, steroids, and monoclonal antibodies, can

E. M. AlEdani (✉)
University of Basrah-Medical Faculty, Basrah, Iraq

E. M. AlEdani, H. Maibach (eds.), *COVID-19 Vaccination and Dermatological Diseases*, Updates in Clinical Dermatology, https://doi.org/10.1007/978-3-031-87791-9_10

make it more difficult for the immune system to fight against infections.

Disruption of the skin barrier: Prolonged inflammation of the skin in patients with SS weakens the skin's defenses against infection, increasing the risk of secondary bacterial or fungal infections that could worsen COVID-19 results.

Due to their weakened immune systems, patients with SS who get COVID-19 are more likely to experience serious respiratory problems, hospitalization, and death [2].

10.4 Clinical Impact of COVID-19 on SS Patients

10.4.1 COVID-19 Infection Severity

Acute respiratory distress syndrome (ARDS) and severe pneumonia are serious risks that COVID-19 presents to people with sickle cell disease (SS). Chronic inflammation is linked to SS, and this can intensify the cytokine storm observed in severe COVID-19 patients. This raises the possibility of multiple organ failure by starting a hazardous loop of immunological dysregulation.

Furthermore, opportunistic infections are common in SS patients. These individuals' COVID-19 frequently causes fungal or bacterial infections as secondary illnesses, which makes their recovery even more difficult [3].

10.4.2 Disruptions in Treatment and Care

The epidemic has had a serious negative influence on cancer patients' access to healthcare, including SS sufferers. Important difficulties consist of:

Treatments that are delayed or interrupted: Due to lockdowns or patients' concerns about catching COVID-19 in hospital settings, many patients had their chemotherapy or phototherapy sessions cut short.

Clinical trials are not widely accessible to SS patients, who frequently depend on experimental medicines made possible by these trials—many of which were postponed or discontinued during the epidemic.

Limitations of telemedicine: Although virtual consultations have becoming popular, remote care is less effective for SS management since periodic skin inspections and blood testing are necessary.

In several cases, the cumulative impact of these disruptions has caused the disease to advance, which has resulted in worse results [3].

10.5 Vaccination and SS Patients

One of the best defenses against serious COVID-19 consequences is vaccination. Nevertheless, immunizing SS patients presents some challenges:

10.5.1 Vaccine Efficacy in Immunocompromised Patients

Research has demonstrated that people with cancer, particularly those receiving immunosuppressive treatments, respond less well to COVID-19 vaccinations. Patients with SS might not produce enough antibodies following the typical two-dose vaccination course. As a result, health authorities advise:

- **Extra dosages:** To increase immunity, receive a third or even a fourth dosage of mRNA vaccinations.
- **Prevention before exposure**: For patients with impaired immune systems, monoclonal antibodies (like Evusheld) may be advised as a temporary protective measure [4].

10.5.2 Timing of Vaccination with Ongoing Treatment

For SS patients, the timing of vaccinations needs to be carefully coordinated with their treatment regimen. Certain immunosuppressive medications, such monoclonal antibodies or corticosteroids, can reduce the body's immunological response to vaccinations. To optimize vaccination effectiveness, doctors could advise postponing some treatments [4].

10.6 Psychosocial Impact of COVID-19 on SS Patients

In addition to affecting physical health, the pandemic has negatively impacted SS patients' mental health. Psychological anguish is already a result of the chronic nature of SS, and the additional stress of the pandemic has made feelings of melancholy, worry, and isolation worse. Important elements consist of:

Social isolation: Many patients self-isolated to avoid exposure because of their high susceptibility, which resulted in loneliness.

Decreased assistance networks: Patients' access to support networks and caregivers was restricted by hospital lockdowns and other measures.

Treatment uncertainty: Fear and worry regarding the course of the disease were exacerbated by treatment schedule modifications or delays.

During the epidemic, many healthcare providers stressed psychological care in addition to physical therapy, as the need for mental health support became evident [5].

10.7 Lessons Learned and Future Directions

10.7.1 Improved Healthcare Delivery

The epidemic brought home how critical flexible treatment regimens, home-based care, and telemedicine are for those who are particularly vulnerable. Even if it wasn't a perfect solution, these advances made sure that some patients got care in spite of the difficulties brought on by COVID-19 [6].

10.7.2 Continued Vaccination Efforts

For SS sufferers, ongoing immunization campaigns are still essential. Scientists are developing vaccinations of the next generation that may provide immunocompromised people with more comprehensive and durable protection [6].

10.7.3 Long-term Monitoring for COVID-19 Impact

Extended COVID-19, which is defined by enduring symptoms after an acute infection, may present particular difficulties for those with SS. Research and monitoring must be done continuously in order to determine the duration of COVID's interaction with SS and to create efficient management plans [6].

10.8 Conclusion

Patients with Sézary syndrome have experienced significant effects with COVID-19, which have made their underlying immunological dysfunction worse. The epidemic has worsened mental health, interrupted vital medical care, and raised the risk of serious illness. But there has been some respite thanks to immunization programs and advancements in medical care delivery. Developing more specialized vaccinations and treatment plans for immunocompromised individuals will be essential in the future to guarantee them access to complete care even in times of public health emergency.

References

1. Levy Yurkovski I, Rokach L, Melamed G, Alapi H, Gazit S, Patalon T, Tadmor T. Clinical outcomes of COVID-19 in mycosis fungoides and sezary syndrome. Acta Haematol. 2023;146(6):497–504. https://doi.org/10.1159/000531831. Epub 2023 Jul 29. PMID: 37517402; PMCID: PMC11251663.
2. Aram K, Patil A, Goldust M, Rajabi F. COVID-19 and exacerbation of dermatological diseases: a review of the available literature. Dermatol Ther. 2021;34(6):e15113. https://doi.org/10.1111/dth.15113. Epub 2021 Sep 7. PMID: 34453380; PMCID: PMC8646294.
3. Snowden C, Ng S, Choi J. Partial remission of advanced untreated Sézary syndrome after COVID-19. JAAD Case Rep. 2022;21:165–8. https://doi.org/10.1016/j.jdcr.2021.12.005. Epub 2022 Jan 6. PMID: 35013712; PMCID: PMC8734171.
4. Gonzaga Y, Santos MBF, Silva MM, Nucci M. COVID-19 infection in patients with Sézary syndrome: report of two cases. Dermatol Ther. 2020;33(6):e14042. https://doi.org/10.1111/dth.14042. Epub 2020 Aug 13. PMID: 32700814; PMCID: PMC7404374.
5. Chang C, Ristuccia R, Zheng Z, Takahashi T, Nomura T, Dennis E. Real-world use of mogamulizumab among patients with mycosis fungoides and sézary syndrome before and during COVID-19 in the United States. Clin Ther. 2024:S0149-2918(24)00275-3. https://doi.org/10.1016/j.clinthera.2024.09.011. Epub ahead of print. PMID: 39379224.
6. Hernández-Coronado M, Gómez-Almaguer D, Jaime-Pérez JC. Haploidentical hematopoietic cell transplantation for mycosis fungoides/Sezary syndrome using reduced intensity conditioning after brentuximab therapy discontinuation: advantages of an outpatient program in the times of COVID-19. Hematol Transfus Cell Ther. 2021;43(3):357–60. https://doi.org/10.1016/j.htct.2021.05.005. Epub 2021 Jun 21. PMID: 34253503; PMCID: PMC8446262.

The Role of Teledermatology in the COVID-19 Pandemic

11

N. L. Swathi and Esraa M. AlEdani

11.1 Introduction to Teledermatology and COVID-19

The COVID-19 pandemic substantially expedited the implementation of teledermatology, improving accessibility and satisfaction for both patients and providers. Notwithstanding technological and infrastructural obstacles, the transition to teledermatology has demonstrated efficacy in diagnosing and managing diverse dermatological disorders; however, discrepancies in implementation remain among distinct populations and areas.

The emergence of the COVID-19 pandemic requires swift modifications in healthcare delivery, notably the proliferation of teledermatology. Burshtein et al. [1] performed a systematic review of pediatric teledermatology, demonstrating diagnostic concordance rates between teledermatologists and in-person assessments between 70.1% and 89%. This signifies the strong reliability of teledermatology in pediatric healthcare. Furthermore, patient satisfaction scores ranged from 70% to 98%, while provider satisfaction was approximately 95%, highlighting the favorable reception of teledermatology among both parties.

Yeboah et al. [2] examined the extensive effects of COVID-19 on teledermatology, emphasizing both achievements and limitations. This review highlighted that teledermatology enhanced access to care and mitigated COVID-19 exposure hazards. Nonetheless, constraints such as image quality and inability to conduct thorough skin assessments are prevalent issues. Shah et al. [3] validated these findings, indicating that 64% of the surveyed academic dermatologists regarded teledermatology as effective for patient care due to enhanced access and convenience, while 37% associated its implementation with professional burnout, primarily due to technical challenges and image quality concerns.

In specialized contexts, Curr Dermatol Rep. [4] assessed inpatient teledermatology and determined that its implementation during the pandemic was equivalent to in-person evaluations of triage and management of diverse disorders. Notwithstanding its cost-effectiveness, obstacles to reimbursement impede its extensive implementation. Likewise, J Med Internet Res [5]. evaluated asynchronous electronic communication visits, such as teledermatology, and discovered that, although clinical outcomes frequently paralleled those of in-person visits, the quality of care exhibited variability, especially in infection management situations.

N. L. Swathi (✉)
Department of Pharmacy Practice, Jawaharlal Nehru Technological University,
Anantapur, Andhra Pradesh, India

E. M. AlEdani
University of Basrah-Medical Faculty, Basrah, Iraq

E. M. AlEdani, H. Maibach (eds.), *COVID-19 Vaccination and Dermatological Diseases*, Updates in Clinical Dermatology, https://doi.org/10.1007/978-3-031-87791-9_11

Pathog Glob Health. [6] investigated telemedicine adoption among Asian-Americans during the epidemic, highlighting lower adoption rates relative to other demographics. This gap was ascribed to technological obstacles and diminished healthcare understanding connected to COVID-19 among this cohort. [7] examined treatment adherence in dermatology during COVID-19 and discovered that excellent communication via telemedicine markedly enhanced adherence rates, notwithstanding apprehensions regarding infection risk linked to immunomodulatory therapies.

JMIR Dermatol. [8] offers an additional layer of analysis of the efficacy of store-and-forward (SAF) teledermatology. The research showed that photographs submitted by clinicians resulted in superior diagnostic accuracy relative to those submitted by patients, highlighting the significance of skilled professionals in image acquisition. This differentiation is essential for streamlining teledermatological processes and improving the diagnostic accuracy.

Finally, Dermatol Online J. [4] concentrated on patient safety in dermatology, encompassing telemedicine elements. The analysis emphasized that although teledermatology reduces physical contact and potential COVID-19 exposure, it raises new safety concerns, including data security and accuracy of diagnoses without in-person examinations. This highlights the need for stringent rules and training to alleviate the dangers of virtual consultations.

Cumulative evidence highlights that the COVID-19 pandemic accelerated the extensive implementation of teledermatology, showcasing its effectiveness and elevated satisfaction levels. Nonetheless, obstacles include technological limitations, variability in image quality, and persistent differences in adoption among diverse populations. The evidence quality, predominantly Level IV, owing to observational study designs, indicates the necessity for additional stringent, controlled investigations to better substantiate the usefulness of teledermatology and overcome current constraints.

The COVID-19 pandemic accelerated the swift incorporation of teledermatology into clinical practice, fulfilling the pressing demand for remote healthcare options. The efficacy and security of teledermatology were demonstrated by heightened satisfaction among patients and providers with the preservation of treatment compliance. However, the transition encountered obstacles. Technological obstacles, including insufficient image quality and technical challenges, have hindered uninterrupted care provision. Moreover, variations in teledermatology use among various ethnic groups, particularly Asian Americans, underscore persistent inequities in healthcare access.

11.2 Teledermatology's Role in Maintaining Dermatologic Care

Teledermatology successfully maintained the continuity of dermatological care during lockdowns by remotely addressing numerous chronic skin problems, including psoriasis, severe acne, atopic dermatitis, hidradenitis suppurativa, and blistering autoimmune illnesses. Furthermore, psychosocial teleconsultations and telementoring programs, such as Dermatology ECHO, have augmented patient quality of life and facilitated access to specialized dermatological expertise in underserved areas.

The adoption of teledermatology during lockdowns has proven essential in ensuring the continuity of care for patients with chronic dermatological problems. Brunasso and Massone (2020) documented the implementation of a teledermatology service in Italy during the COVID-19 shutdown and effectively remotely monitored 183 of 195 patients [9]. The controlled conditions comprised 126 cases of moderate to severe psoriasis, 10 cases of severe acne, 11 cases of severe atopic dermatitis, 11 cases of hidradenitis suppurativa, 9 cases of blistering autoimmune illnesses, and 16 cases of other autoimmune skin disorders. Significantly, only 2.7% (five patients) required in-person visits, reflecting a considerable decrease in face-to-face consultations. This study highlights the effectiveness of teledermatology in preventing illness exacerbation and guaranteeing treatment adherence, although it is constrained by its observational methodology and the absence of a control group, potentially affecting the generalizability of the results.

Marasca et al. (2022) broadened the domain of teledermatology by integrating psychological teleconsultations to mitigate the emotional effects of chronic skin conditions during the pandemic [10]. Their service conducted 23 psychological video consultations, leading to a notable reduction in the Dermatology Life Quality Index (DLQI) from 4.4 ± 3.9 at baseline to 1.6 ± 2.5 by week four. This quantitative enhancement underscores the capacity of integrated teledermatology services to improve both the clinical results and patients' psychological well-being. The limited sample size and brief follow-up duration undermine the reliability of these conclusions, requiring larger longitudinal research to corroborate these findings.

Lewis et al. (2018) presented the Dermatology Extension for Community Healthcare Outcomes (ECHO) project as a telementoring initiative designed to mitigate the scarcity of dermatologists in rural and underserved regions [11]. This study utilized multidisciplinary case-based telementoring and continuing medical education (CME) to enable primary care practitioners (PCPs) to handle intricate dermatologic disorders. The authors demonstrated its impact through a case study of a 69-year-old woman who experienced substantial clinical improvement following the discussion of her case in a Dermatology ECHO session. This narrative illustrates the practical advantages of the ECHO model; however, it mostly represents an expert view and lacks empirical evidence to validate its effectiveness in larger populations.

These studies collectively demonstrate the efficacy of teledermatology in ensuring the continuity of care during lockdowns. Quantitative data from Brunasso and Massone [9] and Marasca et al. [10] provide measurable outcomes; however, they are constrained by methodological restrictions, including small sample numbers and observational designs. Lewis et al. [11], although less empirical, contributed a significant perspective by examining systemic access challenges via telementoring. The disparity in evidence levels among these studies underscores the necessity for more rigorous controlled research to thoroughly assess the impact and scalability of teledermatology.

The examined literature demonstrates that Teledermatology is an essential tool for maintaining the continuity of dermatologic care during lockdowns, efficiently addressing a range of chronic skin disorders remotely. Brunasso and Massone's (2020) findings in Italy illustrate teledermatology's efficacy in managing substantial patient loads with few face-to-face interactions, consequently diminishing the likelihood of illness aggravation and promoting treatment adherence [9]. Marasca et al. (2022) substantiate these findings by demonstrating the supplementary advantages of psychological assistance via teleconsultations, which markedly enhanced patients' quality of life [10]. The Dermatology ECHO initiative, as articulated by Lewis et al. (2018), underscores the strategic significance of telementoring in disseminating specialized dermatological knowledge to impoverished areas, thus alleviating disparities in access to care [11].

11.3 Technological Advancements in Teledermatology

Incorporating mobile health artificial intelligence (AI) into teledermatology techniques augments diagnostic precision, boosts patient accessibility, and optimizes data management using electronic health records (EHRs). The literature indicates that AI-driven mobile health solutions enhance the early detection of dermatological disorders, streamline clinical workflows, and promote tailored patient care, notwithstanding the limitations associated with data integration and technological adoption.

The incorporation of mobile health AI in teledermatology is complex and involves diagnostic improvements, data administration, and the optimization of patient care. Perrone et al. [12] underscored the crucial function of AI in telemedicine throughout the Covid-19 pandemic, particularly its use in teledermatology for prompt identification and diagnosis of cutaneous manifestations. This research highlights that AI-driven mobile health systems can decrease the necessity for in-person clinical appointments, thus reducing exposure risks and ensuring continuity of service. This is consistent with Zhao et al. [13], who showed that convolutional neural networks (CNNs) attained an area under the curve (AUC) of 0.981 ± 0.015 in psoriasis diagnosis, exceeding the accuracy of 25 Chinese dermatologists, with the AUC not directly compared but suggesting superior performance owing to lower misdiagnosis rates.

Bergier et al. [14] examined the incorporation of big data and intelligent technologies into digital health systems, specifically for the management of systemic autoimmune disorders. The principles discussed, while not solely centered on teledermatology, are applicable, indicating that the incorporation of AI into EHRs improves data-driven decision-making and patient surveillance. AI's capacity of AI to evaluate extensive datasets can facilitate more nuanced and tailored treatment strategies, which is vital in chronic dermatological disorders where patient compliance and long-term care are crucial.

Despite being written in 2000, Stanberry [15] offers essential insights into the challenges and prospects of telemedicine, particularly in teledermatology. This essay delineates the operational, ethical, and regulatory issues that continue to impede the integration of AI and EHRs within teledermatology. Notwithstanding the progress made since 2000, challenges including data protection, interoperability of electronic records, and the necessity for standardized protocols persist. Stanberry's historical viewpoint highlights the necessity of confronting these obstacles to maximize the potential of AI in teledermatology.

Zhao et al. [13] provided substantial evidence for AI efficacy by utilizing a comprehensive dataset of 8,021 clinical images and a diagnostic comparison of 100 images. The substantial decrease in misdiagnosis rates from 0.10 to 0.04 illustrates AI's capacity of AI to improve diagnostic accuracy. Perrone et al. [12] asserted that AI functionalities in EHRs enhance the analysis of patient data, allowing for real-time monitoring and treatment modifications, which are essential during public health emergencies such as the Covid-19 outbreak.

Bergier et al. [14] warned that the scalability and cost-effectiveness of AI systems in electronic health records presents significant obstacles. The incorporation of AI into current health information systems necessitates considerable investment and technological infrastructure, which may not be consistently accessible across different healthcare environments. The reliability of AI algorithms is contingent upon the quality and diversity of the input data, requiring ongoing updates and validation across varied patient populations to mitigate biases and guarantee equitable care.

The synthesis of the examined literature unequivocally demonstrates that the incorporation of mobile health AI into teledermatology practices and electronic health records provides substantial advantages in diagnostic precision, patient accessibility, and data management efficacy. AI-driven techniques, especially convolutional neural networks (CNNs), have exhibited enhanced efficacy in diagnosing dermatological disorders, such as psoriasis, as reported by Zhao et al. [13]. These breakthroughs have enabled early detection and diminished reliance on limited dermatology specialists, particularly in underserved areas. Moreover, the implementation of AI in EHRs, as examined by Perrone et al. [12] and Bergier et al. [14], augments the ability to analyze extensive patient data, facilitates tailored treatment strategies, and enhances patient outcomes.

However, the integration process presents challenges. The ethical problems of patient data protection, necessity for interoperable systems, and possibility of algorithmic biases must be thoroughly addressed. Stanberry [15] identified historical constraints that continue to be pertinent, emphasizing the need for strong legal frameworks and defined standards to regulate AI applications in teledermatology. Furthermore, it is imperative to guarantee the scalability and cost efficiency of AI technologies to avert inequalities in healthcare provision.

11.4 Clinical Outcomes and Limitations (Table 11.1)

Table 11.1 Diagnostic accuracy and limitations of teledermatology vs. in-person dermatology

Aspect	Teledermatology	In-person dermatology	Source
Diagnostic accuracy	Sensitivity of teledermatology in diagnosing skin cancer ranges from 59% to 100% depending on the lesion type, with specificity between 30% and 100% depending on diagnostic thresholds and lesion types	In-person diagnosis sensitivity for skin cancer typically between 67% and 85%	Cochrane review of 22 studies; BMJ systematic review [16, 17]
Accuracy for common conditions	For non-cancerous dermatologic conditions, accuracy in teledermatology is high, with diagnostic agreement between 51% and 85%	Higher diagnostic reliability, particularly for more complex conditions or in-person biopsy and tests	American Journal of Clinical Dermatology [18]
Complex cases	Teledermatology faces challenges with complex, rare, or atypical conditions, which may require in-person examination or additional testing like biopsies	Better suited for complex or unusual presentations due to physical exams, direct imaging, and biopsies	Review during COVID-19 pandemic shows need for in-person follow-up [16, 18]
Technological limitations	Dependent on image quality and the ability of non-dermatologist practitioners to capture adequate photos. Diagnostic outcomes improve with high-quality images and dermatoscopy	Immediate access to all diagnostic tools, including biopsies and high-resolution imaging	Cochrane review on diagnostic limitations [17]

11.5 Patient and Provider Perspectives

Patient satisfaction, ease of use, and access challenges.

Teledermatology markedly improved patient satisfaction during the COVID-19 pandemic, especially in the pediatric population. Consistently high satisfaction rates were observed; however, technological issues, particularly in marginalized communities, remained prevalent.

The influence of teledermatology on patient satisfaction during the COVID-19 pandemic has been significantly favorable, as demonstrated in previous publications. Burshtein et al. (1)performed a thorough systematic review of pediatric teledermatology, analyzing 44 publications published from 2008 to 2022. The analysis demonstrated that the diagnostic agreement between pediatric teledermatologists and in-person dermatologists varied from 70.1% to 89%, signifying a substantial degree of diagnostic reliability in teledermatology services. Patient satisfaction with teledermatology ranges from 70% to 98%, and provider satisfaction remains at approximately 95% [1]. These findings indicate that teledermatology not only preserves but may also improve patient and physician satisfaction compared to conventional in-person consultations.

Furthermore, the study emphasized that teledermatology significantly lowered missed appointments and wait times, which are essential elements influencing total patient satisfaction. The capacity to deliver care remotely has proven especially advantageous during the epidemic, decreasing the necessity for patient travel, thereby mitigating the danger of SARS-CoV-2 transmission. Nevertheless, the analysis highlighted substantial technological obstacles that impede the extensive implementation of teledermatology, particularly in marginalized groups. Challenges include restricted access to high-speed Internet, insufficient digital literacy among patients, and inadequate infrastructure to facilitate teledermatology platforms [1].

Conversely, the analysis of Daneshpazhooh and Mahmoudi [19] offers contextual insight into the teledermatology framework in Iran during the COVID-19 pandemic. This article does not measure patient satisfaction, but highlights the swift adaptation of dermatological techniques to teledermatology due to pandemic-related constraints. The authors examined the integration of teleder-

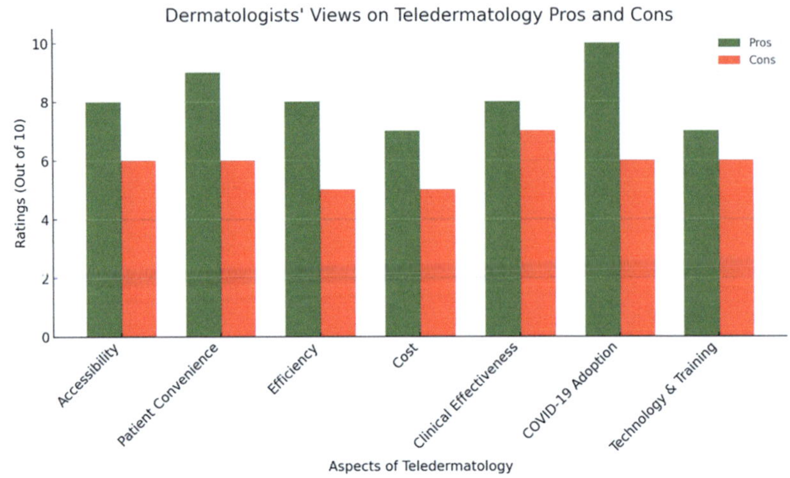

Fig. 11.1 Dermatologists' views on teledermatology's pros and cons. [18, 20–22]

matology by Iranian dermatologists to provide continuity of service, emphasizing the associated opportunities and limitations. The transition to teledermatology is crucial in guaranteeing that patients maintain access to essential dermatological care without disruption, thus indirectly enhancing patient satisfaction through continuous service availability [19].

The paucity of studies examining the influence of teledermatology on patient satisfaction reveals a gap in the literature. The current data are primarily from centers on pediatric populations, as demonstrated by Burshtein et al. [1], which may not adequately reflect the experiences of the wider adult patient demographics. Furthermore, the discovered technological hurdles indicate that, although patient satisfaction is elevated among individuals who can utilize teledermatology services, there exists a segment of the population for whom these services are less accessible or efficacious. This gap necessitates focused initiatives to improve the teledermatology infrastructure and digital literacy, especially in underprivileged areas, to guarantee equal patient satisfaction among various demographic groups.

The elevated provider satisfaction documented in this systematic review signifies the feasibility of teledermatology as a sustainable healthcare delivery method. Providers value the adaptability and efficacy of teledermatology, which can enhance workflow and diminish burnout, elements that indirectly enhance patient satisfaction by improving provider performance and availability. Nonetheless, input from Iran underscores the imperative for sustained support and resources to tackle the operational problems of teledermatology, including data privacy assurance, financing acquisition for telehealth infrastructure, and training provision for healthcare personnel [1].

The integration of the existing literature indicates that teledermatology has been helpful in maintaining and even improving patient satisfaction during the COVID-19 pandemic. A comprehensive review by Burshtein et al. [1] presents compelling evidence of elevated satisfaction rates among pediatric patients, corroborated by dependable diagnostic results akin to in-person consultations. This indicates that teledermatology is not only an effective alternative, but also a favored option for several patients, providing convenience and alleviating obstacles linked to conventional healthcare appointments (Fig. 11.1).

11.6 Policy and Regulatory Changes

This table highlights the various policy shifts that helped teledermatology thrive during the pandemic, facilitating wider access and affordability for patients while also encouraging healthcare providers to adopt telemedicine practices (Table 11.2).

Table 11.2 Policy and regulatory changes supporting teledermatology during the COVID-19 pandemic

Policy/regulatory change	Description	Impact on teledermatology	References
Relaxation of state licensure requirements	Temporary waivers allowed dermatologists to practice telemedicine across state lines without needing additional licenses	Increased access to dermatology care for patients in underserved areas or those with limited local specialists	[20, 22]
Payment parity for telemedicine	Several states mandated payment parity, requiring insurers to reimburse telemedicine at the same rate as in-person visits	Ensured financial sustainability for providers, encouraging the rapid adoption of teledermatology services	[21]
Expansion of medicare telehealth services	Medicare temporarily covered teledermatology services across all locations (including homes), and for a broader set of services, not limited to rural areas	Expanded teledermatology access, particularly for elderly patients and those in remote locations	[22]
Coverage of audio-only consultations	In 18 states, regulations were introduced to cover teledermatology via phone consultations, which previously were not billable	Increased access for patients without reliable internet or familiarity with video technology, especially older adults	[21]
Elimination of patient cost-sharing	Some states and insurers reduced or eliminated co-pays for telehealth services, including teledermatology, during the pandemic	Made teledermatology more affordable, leading to increased patient use, particularly among low-income populations	[21]
HIPAA enforcement discretion	Temporarily, healthcare providers could use non-compliant platforms like Zoom or Skype for teledermatology without penalties	Allowed quick setup and accessibility of teledermatology services using widely available technology during the pandemic	[22]
Extension of reimbursement flexibility	CMS extended the ability to bill for store-and-forward (asynchronous) teledermatology, which is typically used in dermatology for reviewing images sent by patients	Improved efficiency, as dermatologists could review cases without needing real-time interaction, reducing appointment backlogs	[20, 22]

11.7 Conclusion

Teledermatology has played a crucial role during the COVID-19 pandemic by providing effective diagnostics and management of various dermatological conditions. However, its success depends on quality, with clinician-submitted images providing superior diagnostic accuracy. Standardized practices are essential for ensuring equitable access across diverse populations. The pandemic has transformed teledermatology, but the current data lack rigorous research and geographic concentration. Telementoring programs, such as Dermatology ECHO, enhance primary care clinicians' capabilities and broaden access to dermatologic treatment. Integrating mobile health AI with teledermatology offers enhanced diagnostic capabilities and streamlined patient management. However, successful implementation requires overcoming barriers related to technological integration, data privacy, and ethical standards. Future research should expand the scope of the studies to include diverse patient demographics and geographic regions. To fully realize the benefits of teledermatology, concerted efforts are needed to address technological challenges and ensure equitable access to services.

References

1. Burshtein J, Buethe MG, Ghias MH, Stein AB, Glick S, Marmon S. Efficacy, perception, and utilization of pediatric teledermatology: a systematic review. JAAD Int. 2023;12:3–11.
2. Yeboah CB, Harvey N, Krishnan R, Lipoff JB. The impact of COVID-19 on teledermatology: a review. Dermatol Clin. 2021;39(4):599–608.
3. Shah P, Dorrell DN, Feldman SR, Huang WW. The impact of teledermatology during the COVID-19 pandemic. Dermatol Online J. 2021;27(10).

4. Mocharnuk J, Lockard T, Georgesen C, English JC. Inpatient teledermatology: a review. Curr Dermatol Rep. 2022;11(2):52–9.
5. Nguyen OT, Alishahi Tabriz A, Huo J, Hanna K, Shea CM, Turner K. Impact of asynchronous electronic communication-based visits on clinical outcomes and health care delivery: systematic review. J Med Internet Res. 2021;23(5):e27531.
6. Anand S, Cao E, Kimura R, Guo W, Bassi N. Asian American vaccination, testing, and other healthcare knowledge & behaviors during COVID-19, a systematic review. Pathog Glob Health. 2023;117(2):120–33.
7. Bridgeman SG, Perche PO, Feldman SR. Treatment adherence in dermatology during the COVID-19 pandemic: a review. Cureus. 2023;15(1):e34141.
8. Jiang SW, Flynn MS, Kwock JT, Nicholas MW. Store-and-forward images in teledermatology: narrative literature review. JMIR Dermatol. 2022;5(3):e37517.
9. Brunasso AMG, Massone C. Teledermatologic monitoring for chronic cutaneous autoimmune diseases with smartworking during COVID-19 emergency in a tertiary center in Italy. Dermatol Ther. 2020;33(4):e13495.
10. Marasca C, De Rosa A, Fabbrocini G, Cantelli M, Patrì A, Vastarella M, et al. Psychological teleconsultations in patients suffering from chronic skin diseases during the COVID-19 era: a service to improve patients' quality of life. J Dermatol Treat. 2022;33(3):1736–7.
11. Lewis H, Becevic M, Myers D, Helming D, Mutrux R, Fleming D, et al. Dermatology ECHO—an innovative solution to address limited access to dermatology expertise. Rural Remote Health. 2018;18(1):4415.
12. Perrone G, Bilotta C, Tullio V, Pirrone R, Argo A, Zerbo S. Telehealth modulation and new proposals during the Covid-19 pandemic: a literature review. Clin Ter. 2022;173(5):489–95.
13. Zhao S, Xie B, Li Y, Zhao X, Kuang Y, Su J, et al. Smart identification of psoriasis by images using convolutional neural networks: a case study in China. J Eur Acad Dermatol Venereol JEADV. 2020;34(3):518–24.
14. Bergier H, Duron L, Sordet C, Kawka L, Schlencker A, Chasset F, et al. Digital health, big data and smart technologies for the care of patients with systemic autoimmune diseases: where do we stand? Autoimmun Rev. 2021;20(8):102864.
15. Stanberry B. Telemedicine: barriers and opportunities in the 21st century. J Intern Med. 2000;247(6):615–28.
16. Bourkas AN, Barone N, Bourkas MEC, Mannarino M, Fraser RDJ, Lorincz A, et al. Diagnostic reliability in teledermatology: a systematic review and a meta-analysis. BMJ Open. 2023;13(8):e068207.
17. What is the diagnostic accuracy of teledermatology for the diagnosis of skin cancer in adults? [Internet]. [cited 2024 Oct 7]. Available from: https://www.cochrane.org/CD013193/SKIN_what-diagnostic-accuracy-teledermatology-diagnosis-skin-cancer-adults
18. Hwang JK, del Toro NP, Han G, Oh DH, Tejasvi T, Lipner SR. Review of teledermatology: lessons learned from the COVID-19 pandemic. Am J Clin Dermatol. 2024;25(1):5–14.
19. Daneshpazhooh M, Mahmoudi H. COVID-19: The experience from Iran. Clin Dermatol. 2021;39(1):23–32.
20. Brown Z, Dobry A. Teledermatology lessons during the COVID-19 pandemic. Curr Dermatol Rep. 2023;12(4):155–60.
21. States' Actions to Expand Telemedicine Access During COVID-19 and Future Policy Considerations [Internet]. 2021 [cited 2024 Oct 7]. Available from: https://www.commonwealthfund.org/publications/issue-briefs/2021/jun/states-actions-expand-telemedicine-access-covid-19
22. Stephanie K, Lin BA, Annika M, Deitermann BS, Christopher J, Miller MD, Amit Garg MD, Jonathan Ungar MD, Harrison P, Nguyen MD. Evolving teledermatology policy and reimbursement landscape in the United StatesCapsule Summary. JAAD Int. 2023;11:200–8.

Impact of Covid 19 on Skin Microbiome

12

Shaik Firoz, S. Kavitha, G. Swapna,
Maleehah Faatimah, Md. Ayesha Sultana,
N. L. Swathi, and Esraa M. AlEdani

12.1 Introduction

A wide variety of microorganisms constitute the skin microbiome, which is essential for immune system function, homeostasis, and skin health. The structural and functional significance of this microbiome in skin physiology and general health is highlighted by the fact that dysbiosis is linked to a number of dermatological disorders, including psoriasis and acne.

In recent years, the intricacy of the skin microbiome has attracted considerable attention, highlighting its critical role in dermatological health and illness. In addition to acting as a barrier against infections, the skin also harbors a unique microbiota that is mainly made up of Staphylococcus, Cutibacterium, and other genera that support homeostasis and local immune response [1, 2]. When this microbial population is disturbed, dysbiosis can result, which is frequently seen in diseases such atopic dermatitis, psoriasis, and acne vulgaris [1, 3].

When comparing skin illnesses to healthy individuals, recent systematic reviews show a significant decrease in microbial diversity, with a preponderance of harmful bacteria [1–3]. For instance, Xu and Li (2019) elucidate how the skin microbiome, particularly Cutibacterium acnes, is intimately involved in the pathophysiology of acne by modulating sebum production and inflammatory responses, revealing a clear correlation between specific microbial profiles and disease severity [4]. Additionally, Byrd et al. (2018) stress that the structure-function relationship of the skin microbiome varies greatly, not only between individuals but also across various anatomical skin sites, suggesting the influence of individual host profiles like

S. Firoz (✉)
Sri Venkateswara Pharmacy College,
Chittor, Andhra Pradesh, India

S. Kavitha
Department of Allied Health Sciences, School of Health Sciences, The Apollo University,
Chittor, Andhra Pradesh, India

G. Swapna
Department of Pharmaceutics, Apollo Institute of Pharmaceutical Sciences, The Apollo University,
Chittor, Andhra Pradesh, India

M. Faatimah
Department of Pharmaceutical Sciences,
MRM College of Pharmacy, Jawaharlal Nehru Technological University,
Hyderabad, Telangana, India

M. Ayesha Sultana
Nirmala College of Pharmacy, Autonomous,
Guntur District, Andhra Pradesh, India

N. L. Swathi
Department of Pharmacy Practice,
Jawaharlal Nehru Technological University,
Anantapur, Andhra Pradesh, India

E. M. AlEdani
University of Basrah-Medical Faculty, Basrah, Iraq

E. M. AlEdani, H. Maibach (eds.), *COVID-19 Vaccination and Dermatological Diseases*, Updates in Clinical Dermatology, https://doi.org/10.1007/978-3-031-87791-9_12

genetics and lifestyle as well as local environmental factors [2].

Microbial dysbiosis can affect systemic health, as evidenced by a systematic study that looked at the relationships between the gut and skin microbiota in diseases such hidradenitis suppurativa [1]. This focus on the relationship between the skin microbiome and other microbiomes, such the gut, suggests possible treatment options, such as probiotics and prebiotics, which work to normalize the microbial communities [1, 5].

There are still issues with study methods, especially when evaluating confounding factors like diet, skin care products, and antibiotics that may affect microbial composition, even though the majority of recent research offers strong evidence connecting microbial diversity and richness to skin health [6, 7]. There is also a need for more robust research models that incorporate multi-omics techniques to illuminate causal linkages rather than merely associations, as many reviewed studies frequently rely on small sample sizes or lack rigorous methodological frameworks [8–10].

The investigation of how environmental factors, including air pollution, might cause microbiome imbalances and result in negative health effects adds an intriguing layer [9]. In addition to changing the outermost layer of microorganisms, exposure to toxins can also drive out beneficial species, which can either promote or exacerbate pre-existing skin diseases. Resolving these environmental interactions presents a significant chance to improve our knowledge of skin health and the function of microbiome regulation [9, 11].

The integrity of the skin and immune system depend heavily on the health of the skin microbiome, a dynamic ecosystem. The data clearly show a connection between skin health and microbiome diversity, suggesting that treatments targeted at reestablishing microbial balance may have a major effect on the course of treatment for common skin conditions.

The composition and functional ability of the skin microbiome are critical for preserving skin health and averting dermatological disorders [12–15].

Research indicates that COVID-19 significantly impacts skin health through microbiota dysbiosis, affecting not only the respiratory system but also the skin microbiota. The skin microbiota interacts dynamically with viral infections, rather than acting as an extrinsic barrier, revealing the etiology of skin symptoms and potential prognogenic effects.

A comprehensive review conducted by Franulić et al. [16]. categorized the cutaneous manifestations observed in pediatric populations during the COVID-19 pandemic. The study underscored that personal protective equipment (PPE) usage potentially resulted in microbiome disruption, particularly leading to mask-related acne due to increased colonization of cutaneous pathogens. This aligns with observations of increased acne lesions, which were commonly linked to alterations in skin homeostasis and disrupted microbial equilibrium.

Inchingolo et al. [17] provide foundational insights into the physiological functions of the skin microbiota, reinforcing the significance of maintaining eubiosis in the context of viral infections. Their findings elucidate how dysbiosis might heighten inflammatory responses and compromise skin barrier integrity, exemplifying the complex interplay between cutaneous microbes and the host immune system during COVID-19.

A pivotal empirical study by Zhou et al. [18] explored the consequences of SARS-CoV-2 on skin microbiota, revealing concrete evidence of decreased α-diversity across various body sites, including the skin. Among the 20 studies reanalyzed, a singular study identified a notable downregulation of skin microbiota diversity post-SARS-CoV-2 infection, providing compelling statistical validation ($p < 0.05$). The implications of this dysbiosis on skin health and potential systemic effects warrant further investigation, especially in patients exhibiting skin manifestations of COVID-19.

Ciechanowicz et al. [19] reported on the association of gastrointestinal symptoms with dermal lesions, reinforcing the notion that internal microbiota alterations could manifest as skin symptoms in COVID-19 patients. Of the 441 patients assessed, only a minority presented with dermal symptoms, suggesting that while skin manifestations may be less common, their presence could correlate with gastrointestinal microbiota disruption, representing a crucial area for prospective research.

The examination by Mir et al. [20] contextualizes recent findings within forensic sciences, asserting that modifications in microbial profiles in COVID-19 patients could impede forensic investigations. This perspective introduces an innovative angle to microbiome research by linking alterations to informatic applications, suggesting a wider implication of microbial dysbiosis beyond health into forensic applications.

Baghbani et al. [21] assert that the relationship between viral infections and microbiota is somewhat reciprocal—infected hosts exhibit notable alterations in microbial populations, which could perpetuate a vicious cycle of dysbiosis and compromised immune responses. This indicates a crucial research direction where microbiota modulation might emerge as a therapeutic avenue, especially considering the growing acknowledgment of the microbiome's role in host immunity.

Longitudinal studies reveal a significant correlation between clinical symptoms and microbiota diversity, highlighting the importance of understanding the skin microbiome's role in COVID-19-related dermatological manifestations. This research could inform future microbiome-targeted therapies and patient management strategies, highlighting the need for longitudinal studies to establish cause-effect relationships.

12.2 Mechanisms of Interaction Between COVID-19 and the Skin Microbiome

COVID-19 affects the skin microbiome, leading to dysbiosis and cutaneous manifestations. Mechanisms include viral entry, exacerbating pre-existing conditions, and environmental factors like facemask usage, causing acne and dermatitis. The interaction between COVID-19 and skin microbiome has gained academic attention, with facemask use causing "maskne" due to aerobic bacteria proliferating under masks [22].

Franulić et al. [16] identified direct interactions between SARS-CoV-2 and skin cells that express angiotensin-converting enzyme 2 (ACE2), suggesting a pathway for viral ingress that can lead to widespread inflammatory responses. This inflammatory context is further complicated by the opportunistic growth of pathogenic bacteria when normal skin flora are disrupted, as seen in those wearing masks for prolonged periods. In a comprehensive study, it was indicated that patients with COVID-19 exhibited a reduction in beneficial skin commensals, such as various species of Bifidobacterium, which play a role in maintaining skin health and preventing excessive inflammation [16, 20].

In a broader perspective, Mir et al. [20] highlighted the implications of microbiome dysbiosis on the course of infectious diseases, emphasizing changes in skin microbiota as a facilitating element in the exacerbation of COVID-19-related skin conditions. Notably, the study underscored the increasing prevalence of opportunistic pathogens—a discovery that has significant ramifications for both clinical outcomes and forensic applications. The authors emphasized the necessity for enhanced research into the skin microbiome's alterations during COVID-19, as these changes might provide beneficial insights for managing skin-related manifestations of the disease.

The role of vitamin D3 as documented by Santa et al. [23] resonates considerably within this context, proposing that adequate levels of vitamin D3 may help alleviate some inflammatory responses associated with COVID-19. This is particularly relevant when considering the skin's role in synthesizing vitamin D3, which might influence not just immune responses but also skin health directly, underscoring the interconnectedness of systemic immunity and dermal microbiota during the pandemic.

Further complexity arises from the reduced biodiversity characterized in the skin of COVID-19 patients—specifically, a marked decrease in beneficial strains of Lactobacillus, correlating with heightened inflammatory responses seen in various dermatologic conditions [24]. The findings of Marras et al. [24] suggest that Bifidobacteria may play a fundamental role in stabilizing skin barrier function and moderating immune responses, thus mitigating the severity of skin conditions associated with viral infections. In-depth analyses of patient cohorts revealed altered skin flora diversity in individuals post-COVID-19 infection, with notable increases in pathogenic bacteria.

COVID-19 affects the skin microbiome, leading to dysbiosis and cutaneous manifestations. Mechanisms include viral entry, exacerbating pre-existing conditions, and environmental factors like facemask usage, causing acne and dermatitis. The interaction between COVID-19 and skin microbiome has gained academic attention, with facemask use causing "maskne" due to aerobic bacteria proliferating under masks.

The pathophysiological alterations caused by SARS-CoV-2 have a substantial effect on the skin microbiota; this is especially true for people who have "maskne." Long-term mask use causes microbial dysbiosis and increased occlusiveness, which can exacerbate pre-existing dermatoses and suggest the need for updated dermatological therapy techniques both during and after the pandemic.

The developing notion of "maskne," which was coined to describe acne mechanica caused by prolonged use of face masks, particularly captures the interaction between SARS-CoV-2 infection and changes in the skin microbiota. The use of masks produces a special microenvironment that causes friction, occlusion, and thermal instability, according to Teo's study, which describes the details of mask-induced skin disorders (Teo 2021). Pathogenic bacteria can proliferate and beneficial skin flora can be suppressed in this interacting environment, clearly defining a path to dysbiosis. Increased production of sebum and inflammatory reactions from a variety of skin disorders, such as acne vulgaris and other contact dermatitis problems, might occur from this [25].

In another insightful review by Spigariolo et al., they expand on "maskne" by directly linking prolonged face mask usage to alterations in skin temperature and moisture levels which further aggravate microbial equilibrium on the skin [26]. According to Spigariolo et al., extended textile-skin contact is associated with a higher risk of inflammatory skin diseases, making the link noteworthy. In line with patterns seen in patients suffering from maskne, the authors mention how the application of occlusive barriers altered the skin microbiome, causing virulence factors in organisms like Staphylococcus aureus to be overexpressed.

Moreover, the impact of COVID-19 on the health of neonatal microbiomes has been contemplated, as discussed by Romano-Keeler et al. They emphasize the indirect effects of infection control measures on the microbial colonization during the critical early life period [27]. Limitations on mother-infant interactions, including lower breastfeeding rates among moms with COVID, can have a domino effect on how a baby's microbiota develops, which will ultimately affect how the child's immune system reacts as they grow [27]. Despite focusing mostly on the gut microbiome, this conversation raises questions about the wider ramifications of microbiome research during and after the pandemic, including the skin microbiome.

Lastly, while discussing the complexities of immune responses induced by SARS-CoV-2, Sokolowska et al. provide insights into how systemic inflammation can alter microbiome stability, although their primary focus remains on respiratory systems [28]. The immunological pathways that may be implicated in changing the dynamics of the skin microbiome during viral infections are contextualized by such knowledge. To properly address such significant linkages, a cross-disciplinary strategy in infectious illness and dermatological research may be required to comprehend these pathways.

The SARS-CoV-2 pandemic has significantly impacted the skin microbiome, leading to mask-induced conditions and broader dermatological issues. Disrupted mother-infant interactions in neonates could lead to long-lasting dermatological conditions later in life. The pandemic's dermatological manifestations signal potential changes in microbial communities, requiring tailored interventions and future dermatological practices to incorporate microbiome analysis and management strategies to counteract these challenges effectively.

12.3 Impact of COVID-19-Related Interventions on the Skin Microbiome

The COVID-19 pandemic has led to significant changes in personal hygiene and protective measures, profoundly affecting the skin microbiome. This section examines the impact of these interventions.

(a) **Hygiene Practices**

During the pandemic, increased handwashing and use of alcohol-based hand sanitizers (ABHS) have been crucial for infection control. However, these practices can disrupt the skin's natural microbiome, reducing bacterial diversity and potentially compromising protective functions. Disinfectants and soaps, which contain surfactants and antimicrobial agents, can disrupt the skin's lipid barrier and microbiome, leading to dryness, irritation, and a predisposition to infections. The emulsifying properties of these agents can diminish the skin's natural oils, causing barrier dysfunction [29, 30].

(b) **Prolonged Mask Use (Maskne)**

Mask-wearing can lead to skin conditions like acne and dermatitis due to changes in moisture, friction, and microbial environment. The occlusive nature of masks can disrupt the skin barrier, altering the local microbiome. Prolonged mask use can increase microbial richness and diversity, potentially promoting pathogenic bacteria growth. Mask reuse has been associated with significant bacterial contamination, but further investigation is needed [31, 32].

(c) **Use of Personal Protective Equipment (PPE)**

Extended use of Personal Protective Equipment (PPE) has been linked to skin issues like pressure injuries and contact dermatitis, potentially altering the microbiome. However, the impact of PPE on skin microbiome composition during the COVID-19 pandemic is limited, requiring further research [29].

(d) **Hospitalization and Medical Interventions**

COVID-19 patients receiving intensive medical treatments, including antibiotics and corticosteroids, may experience significant changes in their skin microbiota. Antibiotics can disrupt microbial balance, increasing susceptibility to infections. Corticosteroids may impair skin barrier function and influence microbial communities. Comprehensive studies on these interventions' impact on skin health and microbiome integrity are limited, highlighting the need for future research to develop strategies to mitigate skin-related issues during and beyond the pandemic [29–32].

12.4 COVID-19 and Skin-Related Conditions

Development of New Skin Conditions Linked to COVID-19

COVID-19 has been associated with various skin manifestations and has implications for the microbiome, potentially exacerbating pre-existing skin conditions.

Common Skin Manifestations of COVID-19

1. **Cutaneous Symptoms:**

   COVID-19 can result in a spectrum of skin manifestations, including maculopapular eruptions, urticaria, vesicular rashes, and vascular lesions such as livedo reticularis and retiform purpura [33–38].

   - "COVID toes," characterized by chilblain-like lesions on the toes and fingers, is a notable manifestation frequently reported [33, 34, 36, 39].
   - Morbilliform lesions have been identified as the most common cutaneous sign, often linked to severe COVID-19 cases and higher mortality [38].

Table 12.1 Skin conditions linked to COVID-19: clinical manifestations, microbiome impact, and aggravation of pre-existing conditions

Condition	COVID-19 link	Microbiome impact	Aggravation of pre-existing conditions
COVID toes	Chilblain-like lesions on toes/ fingers [33, 34, 36, 39]	Immune response, endothelial damage [34, 40]	N/A
Maculopapular Rash	Common in moderate cases [33, 35, 37]	Virus-induced damage [34, 40]	N/A
Urticaria	Linked to mild cases [35, 37]	Immune response [34, 40]	N/A
Psoriasis	Exacerbation post-COVID [44–47]	Microbiome disruption [41–43]	Increased severity, new psoriatic arthritis [44–47]
Eczema	Increased cases during the pandemic [30, 48]	Hygiene-related microbiome changes [30, 48]	Aggravation due to microbiome disruption [30, 43]

2. **Mechanisms:**
   - These manifestations are hypothesized to arise from virus-induced endothelial cell damage, immune responses, and microvascular damage [34, 40].
   - Pseudochilblains are associated with an exaggerated IFN-1 production, reflecting immune dysregulation [34].

Changes in the Microbiome Associated with These Conditions

1. **Microbiome Alterations:**
   - COVID-19 significantly alters microbiome composition across body sites, including the skin, gut, and respiratory tract [20, 41, 42].
   - These changes typically feature a depletion of beneficial commensal bacteria and an increase in opportunistic pathogens [41, 42].
2. **Impact on Skin Conditions:**
   - A disrupted microbiome can aggravate skin conditions by impairing the skin's natural defenses.
   - For instance, fecal microbial transplantation (FMT) demonstrated efficacy in alleviating severe eczema linked to post-COVID-19 vaccination, suggesting a strong interplay between microbiome health and skin condition severity [43].

Aggravation of Pre-existing Conditions Like Eczema or Psoriasis

1. **Psoriasis:**
   - COVID-19 has been reported to exacerbate psoriasis, with increased severity and the new onset of psoriatic arthritis post-COVID-19 [44–47].
   - These outcomes may be linked to immune dysregulation and microbiome disruption [20, 41, 42].
2. **Eczema:**
   - An increase in eczema cases has been observed during the pandemic, likely driven by hygiene-related microbiome changes, such as frequent handwashing and sanitizer use [30, 48].
   - The altered skin microbiome compromises the barrier function, aggravating conditions like hand eczema [30, 43, 48] (Table 12.1).

COVID-19 has been linked to diverse new skin conditions and exacerbations of pre-existing conditions like eczema and psoriasis. These outcomes are influenced by immune responses, virus-induced endothelial damage, and microbiome alterations. Treatment strategies, such as fecal microbial transplantation, and optimized skin care are promising avenues for managing these complications. Further investigation is warranted to elucidate the specific mechanisms behind the microbiome's role in aggravating conditions such as eczema and psoriasis.

12.5 Implications of Microbiome Disruption During COVID-19

The COVID-19 pandemic has highlighted the critical role of the human microbiome in health and disease. Disruptions to the microbiome during infection can have significant short-term and long-term consequences, particularly in immune function and susceptibility to other infections.

In the short term, COVID-19 has been associated with substantial alterations in microbiomes across different body niches, including the skin and gut. Skin microbiome changes, marked by an increase in opportunistic pathogens and a decrease in beneficial commensal bacteria, often result in skin irritation and infections [20]. Additionally, the integrity of epithelial barriers, especially in the gastrointestinal tract, is compromised. This disruption exacerbates inflammation and immune dysfunction, weakening the barrier functions that protect against environmental insults and microbial invasion [49, 50].

Long-term microbiome disruption due to COVID-19 presents even greater challenges. Persistent gut dysbiosis has been linked to chronic conditions such as prolonged gastrointestinal disorders, immune deregulation, and delayed viral clearance [51, 52]. Recovery of the gut microbiome after COVID-19 can be slow, with some patients experiencing reduced microbial diversity and ongoing dysbiosis even after clinical recovery. These factors contribute to an increased risk of secondary infections and chronic health issues [52, 53].

Dysbiosis also plays a significant role in immune dysfunction and increased susceptibility to other infections during and after COVID-19. The disruption of the gut microbiome is associated with systemic inflammation and an exaggerated immune response, which is a key factor in disease severity [49, 50, 54]. Gut barrier dysfunction, commonly observed in COVID-19 patients, facilitates the translocation of bacteria into the bloodstream, increasing the risk of life-threatening secondary infections [50]. Furthermore, persistent microbiome alterations have been linked to long COVID, where patients experience prolonged symptoms due to ongoing immune dysregulation and chronic inflammation. Significant changes in the oral and gut microbiomes of these patients may contribute to the persistence of these symptoms [55, 56].

The far-reaching consequences of microbiome disruption underscore the importance of understanding these changes to improve patient outcomes. In the short term, addressing microbiome alterations can help manage immediate complications such as skin infections and reduced barrier integrity. In the long term, therapies targeting microbiome recovery could play a pivotal role in preventing chronic conditions and mitigating the impact of long COVID. Further research is necessary to unravel the complex interactions between SARS-CoV-2 infection and the human microbiome to develop effective therapeutic interventions.

12.6 Strategies to Restore and Protect the Skin Microbiome

The skin microbiome plays a vital role in maintaining skin health, and disruptions can lead to various dermatological issues. This section outlines effective strategies to restore and protect the skin microbiome, focusing on probiotic and prebiotic approaches, optimal skin care practices, innovations in mask design and PPE, and post-COVID rehabilitation interventions.

Probiotic and Prebiotic Approaches
Topical and Oral Therapies:

Probiotics and prebiotics are essential for restoring the balance of the skin microbiome. Probiotics are live microorganisms that confer health benefits when applied topically or ingested, while prebiotics are non-digestible fibers that promote the growth of beneficial bacteria. Topical applications of probiotics, such as formulations containing strains like Lactobacillus and Bifidobacterium, have been shown to enhance skin barrier function and reduce inflammation [57, 58]. Prebiotic ingredients like fructooligosaccharides (FOS) and inulin can also support skin health by nourishing beneficial microbes [59, 60].

Oral probiotics, particularly those derived from fermented foods, can further support the skin microbiome by enhancing gut health, which is closely linked to skin conditions. Regular consumption of fermented products like yogurt, kimchi, and kefir can provide systemic benefits that reflect positively on skin health [59].

Skin Care Practices
Maintaining a Healthy Microbiome:

To maintain a healthy skin microbiome amid increased hygiene practices, it is crucial to adopt gentle cleansing methods. Over-washing or using harsh soaps can strip the skin of its natural oils and beneficial bacteria. It is recommended to use mild, pH-balanced cleansers that respect the skin's natural barrier [57, 60].

Alternatives to harsh sanitizers include alcohol-free hand sanitizers with moisturizing agents or natural oils that do not disrupt the microbiome. Incorporating products with natural ingredients like jojoba oil or green tea extract can also support microbial diversity on the skin [57].

Recommendations for Skin Care:

Use gentle cleansers instead of harsh soaps.

Opt for alcohol-free sanitizers with moisturizing properties.

Include prebiotic and probiotic skincare products in your routine.

Limit exposure to synthetic fabrics and heavy makeup to allow the skin to breathe.

Innovations in Mask Design and PPE
As mask-wearing has become commonplace due to COVID-19, innovations in materials and designs aim to minimize disruption to the skin microbiome. Masks made from breathable fabrics that allow moisture evaporation can help prevent conditions like acne mechanica caused by prolonged mask use. Additionally, incorporating antimicrobial treatments into mask fabrics may help reduce pathogenic bacteria while preserving beneficial microbes [58, 59].

Research into nanotherapeutics is also advancing, with nanoparticle-based systems being developed to deliver probiotics directly onto the skin or modulate microbial communities effectively [60]. Such innovations could play a significant role in maintaining skin health during prolonged use of PPE.

Post-COVID Rehabilitation
For patients experiencing long COVID or lingering effects post-infection, specific interventions targeting microbiome recovery are crucial. This may include tailored skincare regimens incorporating probiotics and prebiotics to restore microbial balance disrupted during illness. Additionally, lifestyle modifications such as a balanced diet rich in antioxidants and fermented foods can support overall recovery [58, 60].

Furthermore, dermatological consultations focusing on individualized treatment plans can help manage any exacerbated skin conditions resulting from COVID-19 infection. Strategies may involve using topical treatments that promote healing and reduce inflammation while enhancing microbiome diversity [57, 60].

Restoring and protecting the skin microbiome involves a multifaceted approach that includes dietary changes, gentle skincare practices, innovative product designs, and targeted interventions for those recovering from COVID-19. By prioritizing these strategies, individuals can enhance their skin health and resilience against various dermatological challenges.

12.7 Research Gaps and Future Directions

Long-Term Microbiome Effects of COVID-19:

Studies show significant changes in the microbiome of COVID-19 patients across various body niches, including the gut, respiratory tract, oral cavity, skin, and vagina. These changes are characterized by increased opportunistic pathogens and decreased beneficial commensal bacteria. The gut microbiome is enriched with opportunistic bacteria, fungi, and eukaryotic viruses, which are associated with disease severity and presentation. These gut microbiome features persist in a significant subset of patients even after disease resolution [61–63].

Interactions Between COVID-19 Therapies and the Microbiome:

The COVID-19 pandemic has highlighted the urgent need for improved probiotic and antibiotic use, with potential causal relationships between gut microbiota and COVID-19. Inflammatory factors mediate this relationship, and while the relationship between COVID-19 severity and the human microbiome remains uncertain, fecal microbiome dysbiosis and increased pathogens have been reported in COVID-19 patients [64–66].

Emerging Tools and Technologies for Studying the Skin Microbiome in the Context of COVID-19:

The COVID-19 pandemic has highlighted the urgent need for improved probiotic and antibiotic use, with potential causal relationships between gut microbiota and COVID-19. Inflammatory factors mediate this relationship, and while the relationship between COVID-19 severity and the human microbiome remains uncertain, fecal microbiome dysbiosis and increased pathogens have been reported in COVID-19 patients [67, 68]

Potential Future Directions for Research on the Skin Microbiome and Its Relationship with COVID-19:

The skin microbiome plays a crucial role in skin disease pathogenesis and progression, and future research will benefit from advancements in technology. The COVID-19 pandemic has significantly impacted gut microbiome research, as it is enriched with opportunistic microorganisms in COVID-19 patients. Accurate investigation of gut microbiota is essential for determining the appropriate microbiome profile for diagnosis and the most reliable antiviral or preventive microbial composition. Current research gaps include understanding the long-term effects of COVID-19, interactions between therapies and the microbiome, emerging tools for studying the skin microbiome, and potential future directions for research on the skin microbiome and its relationship with COVID-19 [62, 67, 69, 70].

12.8 Conclusion

The COVID-19 pandemic has significantly disrupted the skin microbiome, leading to both direct and indirect effects on skin health. Key findings include a reduction in microbial diversity and an increase in pathogenic bacteria across skin sites, contributing to common skin conditions like "COVID toes," acne, urticaria, and exacerbations of pre-existing conditions like eczema and psoriasis. The pandemic-specific phenomena of "maskne" exemplify how environmental and protective measures create microenvironments that disrupt microbial balance and compromise barrier function. Dysbiosis is not limited to the skin but often reflects systemic microbiome alterations. The interplay between the gut and skin microbiota, particularly in conditions like hidradenitis suppurativa and COVID-19-related gastrointestinal symptoms, highlights the interconnectedness of microbiome health across body niches. Interventions targeting microbiome restoration show promise, with probiotics, prebiotics, and innovative dermatological practices emerging as pivotal strategies. However, significant research gaps remain regarding long-term microbiome effects, interactions between COVID-19 therapies and microbial communities, and the efficacy of emerging microbiome-targeted interventions. Advancements in multi-omics technologies and longitudinal studies are crucial for establishing causal relationships and optimizing therapeutic strategies. In conclusion, maintaining microbiome health through tailored interventions and robust research frameworks is essential for mitigating the dermatological and systemic consequences of the pandemic.

References

1. Lelonek E, Bouazzi D, Jemec GBE, Szepietowski JC. Skin and gut microbiome in hidradenitis suppurativa: a systematic review. Biomedicines [Internet]. 2023 [cited 2024 Dec 28];11(8). Available from: http://www.ncbi.nlm.nih.gov/pubmed/37626773
2. Byrd AL, Belkaid Y, Segre JA. The human skin microbiome. Nat Rev Microbiol. 2018;16(3):143–55.

3. Requena T, Velasco M. The human microbiome in sickness and in health. Rev Clin Esp. 2021;221(4):233–40.
4. Xu H, Li H. Acne, the skin microbiome, and antibiotic treatment. Am J Clin Dermatol. 2019;20(3):335–44.
5. Aggarwal N, Kitano S, Puah GRY, Kittelmann S, Hwang IY, Chang MW. Microbiome and human health: current understanding, engineering, and enabling technologies. Chem Rev. 2023;123(1):31–72.
6. Ribet L, Dessalles R, Lesens C, Brusselaers N, Durand Dubief M. Nutritional benefits of sourdoughs: a systematic review. Adv Nutr. 2023;14(1):22–9.
7. Edwards CA, Van Loo-Bouwman CA, Van Diepen JA, Schoemaker MH, Ozanne SE, Venema K, et al. A systematic review of breast milk microbiota composition and the evidence for transfer to and colonisation of the infant gut. Benefic Microbes. 2022;13(5):365–81.
8. Tilley CP, Fu MR, Qiu JM, Comfort C, Crocilla BL, Li Z, et al. The microbiome and metabolome of malignant fungating wounds: a systematic review of the literature from 1995 to 2020. J Wound Ostomy Continence Nurs. 2021;48(2):124–35.
9. Mousavi SE, Delgado-Saborit JM, Adivi A, Pauwels S, Godderis L. Air pollution and endocrine disruptors induce human microbiome imbalances: a systematic review of recent evidence and possible biological mechanisms. Sci Total Environ. 2022;816.
10. Schommer NN, Gallo RL. Structure and function of the human skin microbiome. Trends Microbiol. 2013;21(12):660–8.
11. Boyajian JL, Ghebretatios M, Schaly S, Islam P, Prakash S. Microbiome and human aging: Probiotic and prebiotic potentials in longevity, skin health and cellular senescence. Nutrients. 2021;13(12).
12. Solano F. Metabolism and functions of amino acids in the skin. Adv Exp Med Biol. 2020;1265:187–99.
13. Manos J. The human microbiome in disease and pathology. APMIS. 2022;130(12):690–705.
14. Ventura Spagnolo E, Stassi C, Mondello C, Zerbo S, Milone L, Argo A. Forensic microbiology applications: a systematic review. Legal Med. 2019;(36):73–80.
15. Gilat R, Yazdi AA, Weissman AC, Joyce KM, Bouftas FA, Muth SA, et al. The gut microbiome and joint microbiome show alterations in patients with knee osteoarthritis versus controls: a systematic review. Arthroscopy J Arthroscopic Related Surg. 2024.
16. Franulić D, Parać E, Dolački L, Topalušić I, Lugović-Mihić L. Cutaneous manifestations of the COVID-19 pandemic in schoolchildren and adolescents. Acta Dermatovenerol Alp Pannonica Adriat. 2023;32(4):173–81.
17. Inchingolo AD, Cazzolla AP, Di Cosola M, Greco Lucchina A, Santacroce L, Charitos IA, et al. The integumentary system and its microbiota between health and disease. J Biol Regul Homeost Agents. 2021;35(2):303–22.
18. Zhou J, Yang X, Yang Y, Wei Y, Lu D, Xie Y, et al. Human microbiota dysbiosis after SARS-CoV-2 infection have the potential to predict disease prognosis. BMC Infect Dis. 2023;23(1).
19. Ciechanowicz P, Lewandowski K, Szymańska E, Kaniewska M, Rydzewska GM, Walecka I. Skin and gastrointestinal symptoms in COVID-19. Prz Gastroenterol [Internet]. 2020 [cited 2024 Dec 28];15(4):301–8. Available from: http://www.ncbi.nlm.nih.gov/pubmed/33777269
20. Mir Tul G, Manhas S, Khurshid Wani A, Akhtar N, Shukla S, Prakash A. Alterations in microbiome of COVID-19 patients and its impact on forensic investigations. Sci Justice. 2024;64(1):81–94.
21. Baghbani T, Nikzad H, Azadbakht J, Izadpanah F, Haddad Kashani H. Dual and mutual interaction between microbiota and viral infections: a possible treat for COVID-19. Microb Cell Fact. 2020;19(1).
22. Na HH, Kim S, Kim J, Lee S, Kim Y, Kim SH, et al. Facemask acne attenuation through modulation of indirect microbiome interactions. NPJ Biofilms Microbiomes. 2024;10(1).
23. Santa K, Kumazawa Y, Watanabe K, Nagaoka I. The potential use of vitamin D3 and phytochemicals for their anti-ageing effects. Int J Mol Sci. 2024;25(4).
24. Marras L, Caputo M, Bisicchia S, Soato M, Bertolino G, Vaccaro S, et al. The role of bifidobacteria in predictive and preventive medicine: a focus on eczema and hypercholesterolemia. Microorganisms [Internet]. 2021 [cited 2024 Dec 28];9(4). Available from: http://www.ncbi.nlm.nih.gov/pubmed/33919907
25. Teo WL. The "Maskne" microbiome—pathophysiology and therapeutics. Int J Dermatol. 2021;60(7):799–809.
26. Spigariolo CB, Giacalone S, Nazzaro G. Maskne: the epidemic within the pandemic: from diagnosis to therapy. J Clin Med [Internet]. 2022 [cited 2024 Dec 28];11(3). Available from: http://www.ncbi.nlm.nih.gov/pubmed/35160071
27. Romano-Keeler J, Zhang J, Sun J. COVID-19 and the neonatal microbiome: will the pandemic cost infants their microbes? Gut Microbes. 2021;13(1):1–7.
28. Sokolowska M, Lukasik ZM, Agache I, Akdis CA, Akdis D, Akdis M, et al. Immunology of COVID-19: mechanisms, clinical outcome, diagnostics, and perspectives—a report of the European Academy of Allergy and Clinical Immunology (EAACI). Allergy Eur J Allergy Clin Immunol. 2020;75(10):2445–76.
29. Bhatt S, Patel A, Kesselman MM, Demory ML. Hand sanitizer: stopping the spread of infection at a cost. Cureus. 2024;16(6):e61846.
30. Vindenes HK, Drengenes C, Amin H, Bertelsen RJ. The impact of alcohol-based hand sanitiser and hand washing with soap and water on bacterial skin microbiota composition. JEADV Clin Practice. 2023;2(4):764–74.
31. Merenstein C, Fitzgerald AS, Khatib LA, Graham-Wooten J, Bushman FD, Collman RG. Effects of mask reuse on the oropharyngeal, skin, and mask microbiome. J Infect Dis [Internet]. 2023 [cited 2024 Dec 28];228(4):479. Available from: https://pmc.ncbi.nlm.nih.gov/articles/PMC10428194/

32. Zhong S, Lai Y, Na J, Wu Y. Mask wearing impacts skin barrier function and microbiome profile in sensitive skin. Sci Rep. 2024;14(1):24209.
33. Gramp P, Freeman M. COVID-19 manifestations in the skin. Med Today [Internet]. 2022;23(3):25–8. Available from: https://www.scopus.com/inward/record.uri?eid=2-s2.0-85136198168&partnerID=40&md5=cc622ee6552897a64ad8fb783b50a3cb
34. Brahimi N, Croitoru D, Saidoune F, Zabihi H, Gilliet M, Piguet V. From viral infection to skin affliction: unveiling mechanisms of cutaneous manifestations in COVID-19 and post-COVID conditions. J Investig Dermatol [Internet]. 2024. Available from: https://www.scopus.com/inward/record.uri?eid=2-s2.0-85211738585&doi=10.1016%2fj.jid.2024.03.047&partnerID=40&md5=8986d40cb81650f6801933fb1785522e
35. Ghafoor R, Ali SM, Goldust M. Cutaneous manifestations of Coronavirus Disease 2019. J Cosmet Dermatol [Internet]. 2022;21(9):3667–72. Available from: https://www.scopus.com/inward/record.uri?eid=2-s2.0-85136826552&doi=10.1111%2fjocd.15258&partnerID=40&md5=fce4f7f50e2caa4ada0f48c2c6f12a59
36. Schwartz RA, Lambert WC. COVID-19–specific skin changes related to SARS-CoV-2: Visualizing a monumental public health challenge. Clin Dermatol [Internet]. 2021;39(3):374–9. Available from: https://www.scopus.com/inward/record.uri?eid=2-s2.0-85101883686&doi=10.1016%2fj.clindermatol.2021.01.009&partnerID=40&md5=a5ff6549d84d749e21a15559608e3ab0
37. Gooch MD. A new rash differential: CoVID-19. Adv Emerg Nurs J [Internet]. 2021;43(1):28–34. Available from: https://www.scopus.com/inward/record.uri?eid=2-s2.0-85100534842&doi=10.1097%2fTME.0000000000000336&partnerID=40&md5=b57f267d0756d3329c3b93f96a5acdad
38. Errichetti E, Stinco G. How to differentiate skin rash in COVID, mononucleosis, chickenpox, sixth disease and measles. Curr Opin Infect Dis [Internet]. 2023;36(2):109–13. Available from: https://www.scopus.com/inward/record.uri?eid=2-s2.0-85150218140&doi=10.1097%2fQCO.0000000000000904&partnerID=40&md5=d38ba12583a7566a93986f2ac7883307
39. Koschitzky M, Oyola RR, Lee-Wong M, Abittan B, Silverberg N. Pediatric COVID toes and fingers. Clin Dermatol [Internet]. 2021;39(1):84–91. Available from: https://www.scopus.com/inward/record.uri?eid=2-s2.0-85105495218&doi=10.1016%2fj.clindermatol.2020.12.016&partnerID=40&md5=a645eb6a74745f26cf8e3d5b8e0d9cea
40. Dvoryankova E V, Korsunskaya IM, Slavyanskaya TA. Skin manifestations of COVID-19. RUDN J Med [Internet]. 2021;25(1):9–15. Available from: https://www.scopus.com/inward/record.uri?eid=2-s2.0-85166254034&doi=10.22363%2f2313-0245-2021-25-1-9-15&partnerID=40&md5=620648bdcd14cc4383118dfa6e7f82c6
41. Guha SK, Niyogi S. Microbial dynamics in COVID-19: unraveling the impact of human microbiome on disease susceptibility and therapeutic strategies. Curr Microbiol [Internet]. 2025;82(1). Available from: https://www.scopus.com/inward/record.uri?eid=2-s2.0-85212922453&doi=10.1007%2fs00284-024-04041-9&partnerID=40&md5=5c7a3bd84eaaa8d8cb811f4182e7c04f
42. Pusadkar V, Mazumder A, Azad A, Patil D, Azad RK. Deciphering microbial shifts in the gut and lung microbiomes of COVID-19 patients. Microorganisms [Internet]. 2024;12(6). Available from: https://www.scopus.com/inward/record.uri?eid=2-s2.0-85196909620&doi=10.3390%2fmicroorganisms12061058&partnerID=40&md5=0e099d74aa43f18def27da5291954524
43. Huang T, Lv Y, Wang W, Chen Y, Fan L, Teng Z, et al. Case report: fecal microbiota transplantation for the treatment of generalized eczema occurring after COVID-19 vaccination. Clin Cosmet Investig Dermatol [Internet]. 2024;17:229–35. Available from: https://www.scopus.com/inward/record.uri?eid=2-s2.0-85183833046&doi=10.2147%2fCCID.S443542&partnerID=40&md5=47e7b3e5d5d60eeee5f4e499649cbe7c
44. Katkova K V, Plieva KT, Denisova E V, Zhukova O V, Volnukhin A V, Korsunskaya IM. Influence of coronavirus infection on the course of psoriasis. Meditsinskiy Sovet [Internet]. 2021;2021(12):332–8. Available from: https://www.scopus.com/inward/record.uri?eid=2-s2.0-85115866825&doi=10.21518%2f2079-701X-2021-12-332-338&partnerID=40&md5=d5f335e8677cced32fb3058f36f9468c
45. Zitouni J, Bursztejn AC, Belloni Fortina A, Beauchet A, Di Lernia V, Lesiak A, et al. Children with psoriasis and COVID-19: factors associated with an unfavourable COVID-19 course, and the impact of infection on disease progression (Chi-PsoCov registry). J Eur Acad Dermatol Venereol [Internet]. 2022;36(11):2076–86. Available from: https://www.scopus.com/inward/record.uri?eid=2-s2.0-85133816043&doi=10.1111%2fjdv.18361&partnerID=40&md5=daacd9083739e3dbda68e8718558a0b4
46. Pechatnikova EA, Udzhukhu VY, Artemyeva SI, Plotova UA. Features of the post-COVID course of psoriasis. Klinicheskaya Dermatologiya i Venerologiya [Internet]. 2022;21(5):640–5. Available from: https://www.scopus.com/inward/record.uri?eid=2-s2.0-85141496830&doi=10.17116%2fklinderma202221051640&partnerID=40&md5=58eabd19659e7363e80e68b5abf55877
47. Sukhova TE, Molochkova Y V, Kartashova MG, Karzanov O V. Changes in the clinical course of psoriasis post-COVID-19: a clinical case series. Almanac Clin Med [Internet]. 2021;49(8):550–7. Available from: https://www.scopus.com/inward/record.uri?eid=2-s2.0-

85163030340&doi=10.18786%2f2072-0505-2021-49-065&partnerID=40&md5=57631fbaa0c619e6bd47a9cd090b56d8
48. Goksin S, Imren IG, Cenk H, Kacar N, Duygulu S. The effects of changing lifestyle and daily behaviours in the first months of COVID-19 outbreak on dermatological diseases: retrospective cross-sectional observational study. Turkiye Klinikleri Dermatoloji [Internet]. 2022;32(1):47–55. Available from: https://www.scopus.com/inward/record.uri?eid=2-s2.0-85130717751&doi=10.5336%2fdermato.2021-86574&partnerID=40&md5=a591dedfc4c961bdca3131c49d902d1e
49. Basting CM, Langat R, Broedlow CA, Guerrero CR, Bold TD, Bailey M, et al. SARS-CoV-2 infection is associated with intestinal permeability, systemic inflammation, and microbial dysbiosis in hospitalized patients. Microbiol Spectr. 2024;12(11).
50. Bernard-Raichon L, Venzon M, Klein J, Axelrad JE, Zhang C, Sullivan AP, et al. Gut microbiome dysbiosis in antibiotic-treated COVID-19 patients is associated with microbial translocation and bacteremia. Nat Commun. 2022;13(1):5926.
51. Rossini V, Tolosa-Enguis V, Frances-Cuesta C, Sanz Y. Gut microbiome and anti-viral immunity in COVID-19. Crit Rev Food Sci Nutr. 2024;64(14):4587–602.
52. Zuo T, Wu X, Wen W, Lan P. Gut microbiome alterations in COVID-19. Genomics Proteomics Bioinf. 2021;19(5):679–88.
53. Righi E, Dalla Vecchia I, Auerbach N, Morra M, Górska A, Sciammarella C, et al. Gut microbiome disruption following SARS-CoV-2: a review. Microorganisms. 2024;12(1):131.
54. Martín Giménez VM, Modrego J, Gómez-Garre D, Manucha W, de las Heras N. Gut microbiota dysbiosis in COVID-19: modulation and approaches for prevention and therapy. Int J Mol Sci. 2023;24(15):12249.
55. Haran JP, Bradley E, Zeamer AL, Cincotta L, Salive MC, Dutta P, et al. Inflammation-type dysbiosis of the oral microbiome associates with the duration of COVID-19 symptoms and long COVID. JCI Insight. 2021;6(20).
56. Reyes Z, Stovall MC, Punyamurthula S, Longo M, Maraganore D, Solch-Ottaiano RJ. The impact of gut microbiome and diet on post-acute sequelae of SARS-CoV-2 infection. J Neurol Sci. 2024;467:123295.
57. Skin microbiome: care, restoration, ageing | Vaia [Internet] [cited 2024 Dec 29]. Available from: https://www.vaia.com/en-us/explanations/biology/biological-organisms/skin-microbiome/
58. Haykal D, Cartier H, Dréno B. Dermatological health in the light of skin microbiome evolution. J Cosmet Dermatol. 2024;23(12):3836–46.
59. How to restore your skin microbiome for healthier skin—the science behind skin flora—Boston Derm Advocate [Internet] [cited 2024 Dec 29]. Available from: https://www.bostondermadvocate.com/science-of-skincare/how-to-restore-your-skin-microbiome
60. AL-Smadi K, Leite-Silva VR, Filho NA, Lopes PS, Mohammed Y. Innovative approaches for maintaining and enhancing skin health and managing skin diseases through microbiome-targeted strategies. Antibiotics [Internet]. 2023 [cited 2024 Dec 29];12(12):1698. Available from: https://pmc.ncbi.nlm.nih.gov/articles/PMC10741029/
61. Rossini V, Tolosa-Enguis V, Frances-Cuesta C, Sanz Y. Gut microbiome and anti-viral immunity in COVID-19. Crit Rev Food Sci Nutr [Internet]. 2024;64(14):4587–602. Available from: https://www.scopus.com/inward/record.uri?eid=2-s2.0-85142142632&doi=10.1080%2f10408398.2022.2143476&partnerID=40&md5=74f8b95457c1fe5664d7ba3dc2e8b6fb
62. Brett Finlay B, Amato KR, Azad M, Blaser MJ, Bosch TCG, Chu H, et al. The hygiene hypothesis, the COVID pandemic, and consequences for the human microbiome. Proc Natl Acad Sci U S A [Internet]. 2021;118(6). Available from: https://www.scopus.com/inward/record.uri?eid=2-s2.0-85100227742&doi=10.1073%2fpnas.2010217118&partnerID=40&md5=912f1ea2d76f7e1ab28b05144da524cf
63. Wilson JD, Dworsky-Fried M, Ismail N. Neurodevelopmental implications of COVID-19-induced gut microbiome dysbiosis in pregnant women. J Reprod Immunol [Internet]. 2024;165. Available from: https://www.scopus.com/inward/record.uri?eid=2-s2.0-85198330636&doi=10.1016%2fj.jri.2024.104300&partnerID=40&md5=67ad7a801f48025cf047ef735f500b3b
64. Chattopadhyay I, Shankar EM. SARS-CoV-2-indigenous microbiota nexus: does gut microbiota contribute to inflammation and disease severity in COVID-19? Front Cell Infect Microbiol [Internet]. 2021;11. Available from: https://www.scopus.com/inward/record.uri?eid=2-s2.0-85103082029&doi=10.3389%2ffcimb.2021.590874&partnerID=40&md5=7f162e6d819a96dad19dba55ff9ee67d
65. Lin X, Li YZ, Chen T, Min SH, Wang DF, Ding MM, et al. Effects of wearing personal protective equipment during COVID-19 pandemic on composition and diversity of skin bacteria and fungi of medical workers. J Eur Acad Dermatol Venereol [Internet]. 2022;36(9):1612–22. Available from: https://www.scopus.com/inward/record.uri?eid=2-s2.0-85130291794&doi=10.1111%2fjdv.18216&partnerID=40&md5=d9a9fa7270a42bea75d89615ad855727
66. Zyoud SH, Shakhshir M, Abushanab AS, Koni A, Shahwan M, Jairoun AA, et al. Mapping the output of the global literature on the links between gut microbiota and COVID-19. J Health Popul Nutr [Internet]. 2023;42(1). Available from: https://www.scopus.com/inward/record.uri?eid=2-s2.0-85146485455&doi=10.1186%2fs41043-023-00346-w&partnerID=40&md5=c57a9a49f07d45dfa848a131117fbc62

67. Kong HH, Segre JA. The molecular revolution in cutaneous biology: investigating the skin microbiome. J Investig Dermatol [Internet]. 2017;137(5):e119–22. Available from: https://www.scopus.com/inward/record.uri?eid=2-s2.0-85017545127&doi=10.1016%2fj.jid.2016.07.045&partnerID=40&md5=b2ebac18409481ab85e35123c90c5af3
68. Samaras S, Hoptroff M. The microbiome of healthy skin. In: Skin microbiome handbook: from basic research to product development [Internet]. 2020. p. 3–32. Available from: https://www.scopus.com/inward/record.uri?eid=2-s2.0-85102037764&doi=10.1002%2f9781119593058.ch1&partnerID=40&md5=82701a91912571a3e077927e380c4f97
69. Sehli S, Allali I, Chahboune R, Bakri Y, Al Idrissi N, Hamdi S, et al. Metagenomics approaches to investigate the gut microbiome of COVID-19 patients. Bioinform Biol Insights [Internet]. 2021;15. Available from: https://www.scopus.com/inward/record.uri?eid=2-s2.0-85102426919&doi=10.1177%2f11779322219994 28&partnerID=40&md5=6ca8c1d102b4c0c8ee6b1536466e1c9c
70. Sharma J, Sharma V, Sharma I. the skin metagenomes: insights into involvement of microbes in diseases. In: Metagenomics: techniques, applications, challenges and opportunities [Internet]. 2020. p. 189–98. Available from: https://www.scopus.com/inward/record.uri?eid=2-s2.0-85151180792&doi=10.1007%2f978-981-15-6529-8_12&partnerID=40&md5=6d5f4ddbf6756fd00dddea5012574cee

Index

E. M. AlEdani, H. Maibach (eds.), *COVID-19 Vaccination and Dermatological Diseases*, Updates in Clinical Dermatology, https://doi.org/10.1007/978-3-031-87791-9

MIX
Papier aus verantwortungsvollen Quellen
Paper from responsible sources
FSC® C105338

If you have any concerns about our products,
you can contact us on
ProductSafety@springernature.com

In case Publisher is established outside the EU,
the EU authorized representative is:
Springer Nature Customer Service Center GmbH
Europaplatz 3, 69115 Heidelberg, Germany

Printed by Libri Plureos GmbH
in Hamburg, Germany